Lecture Notes: Orthopaedics and Fractures

Lecture Notes
Orthopaedics and Fractures

T Duckworth

BSc (Hons), MBChB (Hons), FRCS (Eng)
Emeritus Professor of Orthopaedics
University of Sheffield

C M Blundell

MB, ChB, BMedSci (Hons), FRCS (Eng), MD, FRCS (Tr&Orth)
Northern General Hospital
Sheffield, UK

Fourth edition

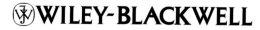

WILEY-BLACKWELL

A John Wiley & Sons, Ltd., Publication

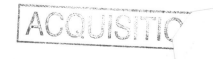

This edition first published 2010, © 2010 by T Duckworth and CM Blundell
Previous editions: 1980, 1984, 1995

Blackwell Publishing was acquired by John Wiley & Sons in February 2007. Blackwell's publishing program has been merged with Wiley's global Scientific, Technical and Medical business to form Wiley-Blackwell.

Registered office: John Wiley & Sons Ltd, The Atrium, Southern Gate, Chichester, West Sussex, PO19 8SQ, UK

Editorial offices: 9600 Garsington Road, Oxford, OX4 2DQ, UK
            The Atrium, Southern Gate, Chichester, West Sussex, PO19 8SQ, UK
            111 River Street, Hoboken, NJ 07030-5774, USA

For details of our global editorial offices, for customer services and for information about how to apply for permission to reuse the copyright material in this book please see our website at www.wiley.com/wiley-blackwell

Library of Congress Cataloging-in-Publication Data
Duckworth, T.
  Lecture notes. Orthopaedics and fractures / T. Duckworth, C.M. Blundell. – 4th ed.
    p. ; cm.
  Rev. ed. of: Lecture notes on orthopaedics and fractures / T. Duckworth. 3rd ed. c1995.
  Includes index.
  ISBN 978-1-4051-3329-6
  1. Orthopedics–Handbooks, manuals, etc. 2. Fractures–Handbooks, manuals, etc. I. Blundell, C. M. (Chris M.)
II. Duckworth, T. Lecture notes on orthopaedics and fractures. III. Title. IV. Title: Orthopaedics and fractures.
  [DNLM: 1. Orthopedic Procedures–Handbooks. 2. Fractures, Bone–Handbooks. WE 39 D836L 2010]
  RD732.5.D83 2010
  616.7–dc22
                              2009046372

ISBN: 9781405133296

A catalogue record for this book is available from the British Library.

Set in 8 on 12 pt Stone Serif by Toppan Best-set Premedia Limited
Printed and bound in Singapore

1 2010

Contents

Contributors

Stephen Bostock
Consultant Orthopaedic Hand Surgeon
Sheffield Orthopaedics Ltd
Sheffield, UK

Ashley Cole
Consultant Orthopaedic Spinal Surgeon
Sheffield Orthopaedics Ltd
Sheffield, UK

Richard Gibson
Consultant Orthopaedic Surgeon
Sheffield Teaching Hospital NHS Trust
Sheffield, UK

Bob Grimer
The Royal Orthopaedic Hospital
Birmingham, UK

Andrew Hamer
Consultant Orthopaedic Surgeon
Sheffield Orthopaedics Ltd
Sheffield, UK

Paul Haslam
Consultant Orthopaedic Surgeon
Doncaster and Bassetlaw Hospitals NHS Trust
Doncaster, UK

Stan Jones
Consultant Orthopaedic Surgeon
Sheffield Orthopaedics Ltd
Sheffield, UK

David Stanley
Consultant Orthopaedic Surgeon
Sheffield Teaching Hospitals NHS Trust
Sheffield, UK

Simon Till
Consultant Rheumatologist
Sheffield Teaching Hospitals NHS Trust
Sheffield, UK

Rob Townsend
Consultant Microbiologist
Department of Microbiology
Northern General Hospital
Sheffield, UK

Preface to fourth edition

Medical training is constantly changing. Surgical training is becoming shorter and the decision about which branch to follow is being asked at an evermore junior level. It is only possible to make an informed career choice by having a sufficient grasp of the relevant speciality and, wherever possible, having some exposure to it.

Orthopaedics is a changing speciality. Sub-specialization has become commonplace and the 'general' orthopaedic surgeon is now rare. This book attempts to introduce most aspects of orthopaedics at a level which will satisfy medical students, students of professions allied to medicine and general practitioners alike.

This fourth edition has been rewritten to make it easier to study the basis of orthopaedics (Part 1) and then to refer to each region in turn (Part 2). With the advent of sub-specialization, this is how the subject is often now encountered. The regional section is further sub-divided into four areas: examination, adult pathology, paediatric pathology and trauma.

We hope we have achieved our goal in creating a book which is broad enough in scope to cover most pathologies whilst covering the more common conditions in sufficient depth to allow a comprehensive understanding.

T Duckworth
C M Blundell

Preface to first edition

At first sight there would appear to be little difficulty in compiling a short textbook of orthopaedics and fractures to meet the needs of medical students, general practitioners and others with a non-specialist interest in the subject. They are all likely to require a quick and reliable source of reference and some practical advice on management. But how much material, how much detail and how much practical advice?

Many medical schools have reduced the time available for the study of disorders of the musculoskeletal system. The medical student is now lucky if he/she can gain experience in the techniques of clinical examination, let alone become familiar with those common orthopaedic conditions which occupy so much of the average general practitioner's time and encroach on every branch of medicine.

It would be a short textbook indeed which covered only the contents of this type of course. Students often complain that they are given no guidance as to how far their reading should take them beyond the confines of their limited clinical experience. They often ask in desperation for a syllabus or a list of reading material: how much do we need to know? Unfortunately, although examiners may be prepared to confine themselves within pre-determined limits, patients rarely do so. They present with obscure problems, or, worse still, common problems in familiar guises. No matter how well he/she has been taught and has understood the principles of diagnosis and management, no textbook can provide the new doctor with what will become his/her most valuable asset—experience. It can however provide him/her with other people's experience and also with something almost equally valuable—an awareness of what are the possibilities. Without this awareness, a diagnosis can rarely be made.

In the absence of clear guidance from the medical faculties about what their end-product, the newly qualified doctor, is supposed to be, it seemed reasonable to try to produce a book which would attempt to provide answers, albeit often brief and incomplete ones, to most of the questions the interested and intelligent student and postgraduate would be likely to ask about the subject.

In doing so, emphasis has been placed on the principles of diagnosis and management and on classification. It is hoped that the latter will be an aid to understanding relationships and also perhaps to memory. Common conditions have been allocated relatively more space, and some details of the management of such conditions, which might be of value to junior staff, are included, with short sections on orthopaedic and operative procedures. Rarities are either excluded or simply receive a brief mention to make the student aware of their existence. Inevitably, some sections will appear too condensed and others too detailed. The section on ankle fractures, for example, is perhaps more appropriate for a trainee orthopaedic surgeon than a student, but here, as in other places, it was felt that the subject could become almost meaningless if less detail was included.

The layout of the book may be found convenient by some readers, irrational and perhaps irritating by others. This particular arrangement has been chosen so that answers will be easy to find, embedded in related information which will make the subject more of a whole. The regional chapters provide an alternative approach to the same information, and cross-references have been provided to avoid repetition.

The content is, of course, the author's choice, based on experience of what has been found useful and of interest to students. Orthopaedics is a strongly clinical subject with a high visual content.

This is reflected in the relatively large number of illustrations. X-rays are so much a part of the world of orthopaedics that it is difficult to imagine the specialty without them, and wherever possible these have been used to illustrate the various conditions. Nevertheless, some experience is required in their interpretation, and where this could be a problem diagrams have been substituted for their extra clarity.

Finally, and in response to suggestions from students, an appendix has been added, giving useful pathological and clinical data for rapid reference.

If this volume proves useful on the wards and in the clinics, and stimulates an interest in a fascinating subject, it may justify adding to the rising tide of published material which threatens to overwhelm students and practising doctors alike.

Part 1

General Principles

Chapter 1

Musculoskeletal structures and function

The skeletal structures

Modern orthopaedics is concerned with the diagnosis and management of disorders of the musculoskeletal system, that is the skeleton and the soft tissues associated with it. Worldwide, orthopaedic surgeons deal with both injuries of the musculoskeletal system, particularly fractures, as well as non-traumatic conditions. Sub-specialization within orthopaedics is increasingly common and can be organized by patient age (e.g. paediatric orthopaedics), by region (e.g. hip surgery) or by condition (e.g. rheumatoid surgery). Alternatively, orthopaedics can be considered in terms of the structures with which it is primarily concerned. A knowledge of the anatomy, physiology and pathology of these structures and tissues forms a logical starting point for studying the clinical aspects of the subject.

The connective tissues

The connective tissues of the body are composed of cells embodied in a matrix which varies in its quantity and composition. The cells can be categorized by the nature of the intercellular material, of which there are three types:

Lecture Notes: Orthopaedics and Fractures, 4e.
By T Duckworth and CM Blundell. Published 2010 by Blackwell Publishing.

- **Bony**—osteoid (produced by osteoblasts)
- **Cartilaginous**—chondroid (produced by chondroblasts)
- **Fibrous**—collagenous tissue (produced by fibroblasts).

Structure

In each case the matrix is mainly composed of a complex mixture of proteoglycans and glycoproteins, forming a ground substance in which is embedded a meshwork of fibrils, mostly of collagen, a protein. At least four genetically different types of collagen are now recognized—bone contains Type I and hyaline cartilage Type II. Skin contains Types I and III and, being a convenient tissue for biopsy, is used for the study of certain collagen-related bone diseases. Elastin, a different protein, is found within skin and to a lesser extent in tendon.

Matrix disorders cause a wide variety of clinical manifestations. For example, in the so-called 'mucopolysaccharoidoses' (see p. 68), an enzyme deficiency interferes with the breakdown of large mucopolysaccharide molecules, which accumulate in the tissues causing widespread abnormalities.

Connective tissues grow by cell proliferation and deposition of intercellular material.

Physiology

The connective tissues are by no means inert and they play an important role in biochemical processes in the body.

Ground substance is an important water-binding agent and acts as an ion-exchange resin in controlling the passage of electrolytes. Its deposition is influenced by many factors, such as hormones and vitamins, and its composition reflects abnormalities in the supply of these factors.

Cartilage 'turnover' is the subject of much research. It is controlled by a complex interaction of different enzymes, some of which promote and others suppress chondrocyte function. Thus, balanced synthesis and degradation of the ground substance has been shown to continue throughout life.

Bone is known to play a vital role in metabolism, mainly because of its calcium and phosphate content. These minerals enter into the formation of crystals of hydroxyapatite and their deposition is sensitive to many influences. Diseases such as rickets, osteomalacia and hyperparathyroidism are associated with dramatic changes in bone development.

Demineralization of bone results in loss of bone strength and may be caused by diminished matrix formation, inadequate calcification or bone resorption. The latter occurs as a result of the activity of special cells—*osteoclasts*—which remove both the organic and inorganic components. The radiographic appearances of loss of density are similar whatever the cause of the demineralization, and these appearances give rise to the term 'osteoporosis', although specific scans (dual energy X-ray absorption [DEXA] scan) are required to make a definitive diagnosis of osteoporosis.

Bone

Macroscopic structure

A long bone is characteristically tubular with expanded ends and is remarkably strong for its weight. The shaft is called the *diaphysis* and the zone adjacent to the epiphyseal line is the *metaphysis* (Fig. 1.1). This is the part of the developing bone that is most likely to be the seat of disease, probably because it is the most metabolically active area and has the greatest blood supply. Damage to, or abnormal development of, the epiphyseal plate itself is likely to result in growth disturbance.

The short bones consist of a cancellous core surrounded by a layer of cortical bone, partly covered by articular cartilage. They contain red marrow in their trabecular spaces and the vertebral bodies are important sites of blood formation throughout life.

A normal bone can resist large compressive forces and considerable bending stresses, and only breaks when subjected to considerable violence. It may, however, be weakened by disease and can then fracture as a result of minimal trauma. Such *pathological fractures* are often orientated transversely across the bone.

The bones form fixed points for muscle attachments and their periosteal sheaths blend with the collagen of the tendons and ligaments.

Microscopic structure

Bone consists of osteoid, which is resilient and is heavily infiltrated with calcium salts, giving it hardness and strength. The mechanism of mineralization is not well understood. The mineral is mainly deposited in crystalline form as hydroxyapatite, but there is also an amorphous phase which is found particularly in newly formed bone. It is worth noting that various ions, such as strontium, fluoride and lead, can enter the crystal lattice of bone mineral.

A normal bone is composed of concentric cylinders of matrix with cells lying in lacunae between the layers, the whole forming a 'Haversian system'. In the hard cortex, the Haversian systems are packed tightly together; in the spongy or cancellous bone, they are more loosely arranged (Fig. 1.2). The bony trabeculae are structured and orientated to withstand the stresses of weight-bearing and muscle activity, obeying Wolff's Law. The interstices of the cancellous bone and the hollow centres of the shafts of long bones are filled with marrow. Haemopoiesis occurs in the marrow throughout the bones in the child, but in the adult is confined to the short bones, particularly the vertebral bodies, and to the ends of the long bones.

Each bone is ensheathed by fibrous periosteum with an underlying layer of osteoblasts, and is

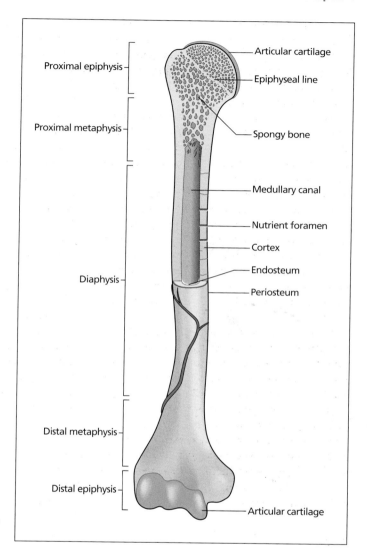

Figure 1.1 Macroscopic structure of bone.

vascularized from the periosteum and by one or more nutrient arteries penetrating the cortex.

Bone formation

The bones develop initially in early intrauterine life as condensations of mesenchymal tissue in the axis of the limb (Fig. 1.3a), and by the sixth week the connective tissue cells have started to lay down cartilage to form the shape of the future bone (Fig. 1.3b). At the centre of the cartilage mass, the cells hypertrophy and apparently die, and with the ingrowth of vascular connective tissue, the matrix calcifies and eventually ossifies (Fig. 1.3c). This process spreads along the bone (Fig. 1.3d), so that it eventually consists of a bony shaft with cartilaginous ends (Fig. 1.3e) which become the sites of secondary ossification centres (Fig. 1.3f). The intervening or epiphyseal cartilage remains until maturity as the growth point for bone length, the proliferating cartilage cells on the diaphyseal side forming into columns and undergoing a series of

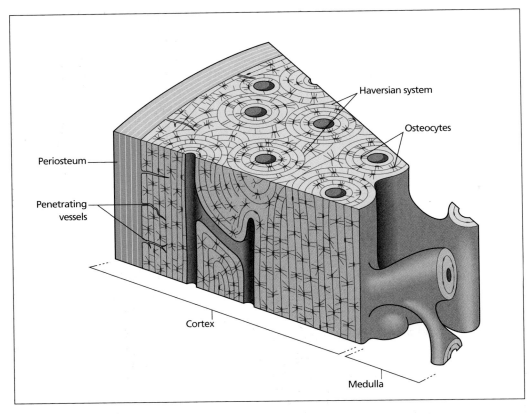

Figure 1.2 Microscopic bone structure.

changes, eventually 'ballooning' as the zone of vascularization reaches them and ossification of the matrix begins. This results in gradual growth of the epiphysis away from the centre of the shaft. Growth in width occurs by deposition of non-cartilaginous subperiosteal bone and the whole bone is constantly remodelled as the child grows.

The earliest bone to be laid down is often called 'woven bone' because its histological structure shows the fibrils to be randomly distributed, unlike the regular lamellar structure of mature bone. Some bones develop entirely by intramembranous ossification, with no intermediate cartilage stage, the clavicle and the skull being examples.

Growth does not occur equally at the two ends of a long bone. It is more active, for example, at the ends farthest from the elbow and nearest to the knee (growth is often described by 'to the elbow I grow, from the knee I flee'). Diseases such as osteo-

myelitis and tumours are noticeably more common at these sites. The spongy ends of the bone have a complex architecture and it is here that the trabeculae can be seen to follow the lines of greatest stress (Fig. 1.4).

Remodelling of bone continues throughout life, but particularly during growth and after fracture healing. In children, even severe residual deformities can be corrected fully, with the possible exception of rotational deformities; this capacity for remodelling is less in the adult and, although the bone smoothes itself out, it is usually possible to spot the site of a fracture many years later (Fig. 1.5).

Cartilage

This varies in appearance and physical characteristics, depending on the predominant type of fibril and the density of the matrix. Two types of fibril,

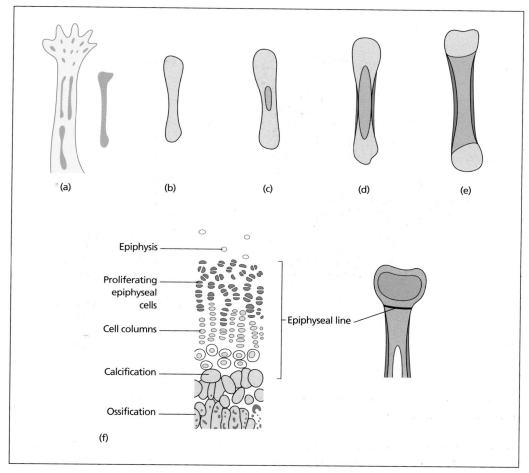

(a) (b) (c) (d) (e)

Epiphysis

Proliferating
epiphyseal
cells

Cell columns

Epiphyseal line

Calcification

Ossification

(f)

Figure 1.3 Bone growth and development.

collagen and elastin, are found in varying proportions. Three types of cartilage are normally recognized.

1 Hyaline cartilage The pre-ossified epiphyses and the articular surfaces both consist of hyaline cartilage, which is indistinguishable in the two by ordinary histological techniques, but has different properties and, of course, different functions in the two tissues.

2 White fibro-cartilage is found mainly in midline structures such as intervertebral discs and symphyses. The collagen content is much greater than in hyaline cartilage and the fibres are much

more obvious. This type of cartilage has the ability to withstand strong tension and bear heavy compressive loads.

3 Yellow or elastic fibro-cartilage is found in the nasal and aural cartilages, and contains the highest proportion of elastin.

Cartilage grows by direct proliferation of the cells with pericellular deposition of matrix, but even during rapid active growth relatively few cells can be seen to be dividing. The capacity of hyaline cartilage to regenerate and repair itself is strictly limited, which means that damage to an articular surface can have long-lasting consequences. There is some evidence that intrinsic mechanisms of repair can be supplemented by ingrowth and metaplasia of periarticular collagenous tissue, but repair of any but the smallest defect is seldom complete.

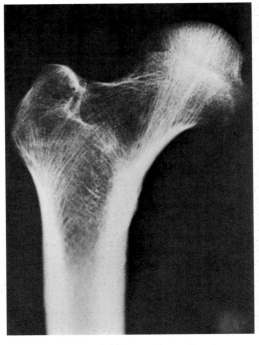

Figure 1.4 Upper end of femur to show trabeculae.

Fibrous tissue

Fibrous tissue is widespread throughout the body and consists mainly of collagen fibres with relatively little matrix.

Disorders of collagen metabolism are being extensively studied because of their dramatic effects on body structure and development. These conditions are sometimes called 'true collagen diseases', as opposed to the non-developmental diseases of collagen, such as rheumatoid arthritis. Osteogenesis imperfecta (see p. 66), is an example of an inherited disorder of collagen metabolism, mainly affecting the structure and strength of bone.

Collagen growth is an important aspect of general body development and fibroblasts are frequently to be seen proliferating and laying down collagen fibres. This is particularly the case in any situation where repair of tissues is required. The usual end-result of repair, the scar, consists almost entirely of collagenous material. In situations where there is continuing damage to the tissues, with concomitant repair, the scar tissue formed can be extremely dense. As it matures, collagenous scar tissue tends to contract, sometimes producing distortion and obstruction of internal structures or contractures of skin and joints. Occasionally, the healing of a skin wound may be complicated

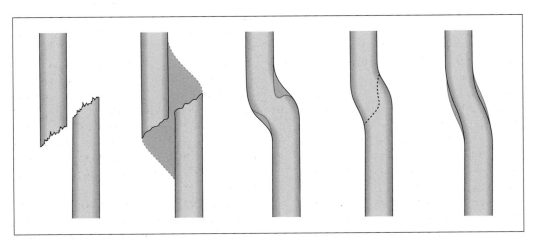

Figure 1.5 Remodelling after a fracture.

by the formation of over-exuberant scar tissue, producing a wide and thickened scar known as 'keloid'. This is more common in races with black skin.

Ligaments

These may be either discrete structures or thickenings of the joint capsule. Being necessary for joint stability, they are strong and are orientated to resist specific stresses. They are, however, occasionally ruptured, either completely or partially, and are difficult to restore when damaged. A partial rupture is known as a *sprain* or *strain*, and usually heals completely.

Joints

The function of a limb is heavily dependent on the smooth working of the joints, and joint diseases are common and troublesome.

Three types of joint are usually recognized.

1 Fibrous joints or syndesmoses. As the name suggests, in this type of joint the bones are connected by a continuous band of fibrous tissue, as is the case with the sutures of the skull. These joints are strong and not readily disrupted, but they allow little movement.

2 Cartilaginous joints or synchondroses. These consist of a cartilaginous band joining the bones. This may be hyaline, as between some of the skull bones, in which case ossification usually occurs at maturity. Secondary cartilaginous joints consist of a mass of fibro-cartilage lying between two thin plates of hyaline cartilage.

3 Synovial joints. This type of joint allows the greatest mobility. The joint surfaces are covered with hyaline cartilage and the joint is enclosed by a fibrous capsule which is usually attached close to the edge of the articular surface. It is lined by a vascular synovial membrane which secretes synovial fluid. This fluid is a remarkable substance which performs a nutritive function and has important lubricating properties. Articular cartilage, apart from its deepest layer, derives most of its nutrition from the synovial fluid which must, therefore,

have access to the whole articular surface. There is some evidence that degenerative joint disease may be, at least partly, due to an interruption in the free flow of this fluid.

Some joints contain fibro-cartilaginous discs partly separating the joint surfaces. The menisci of the knee are examples of this and they have been shown to have an important stress-distributing function.

Articular cartilage, normally smooth and elastic, may be pitted or eroded by disease or completely worn away to reveal the underlying bony cortex. The earliest stages of this process are known as 'fibrillation'. The articular cartilage becomes irregular and tends to fray and split. To some extent, this phenomenon is age-related, but it does not occur uniformly throughout the joints and varies in its extent from individual to individual. It is essentially a focal change, and there are certain sites where it is common, particularly those areas which rarely contact the opposing articular surface and/or where loads are high, such as the patella. In certain circumstances, this condition progresses to fully developed osteoarthritis (see Chapter 11).

Blood supply and innervation of joints

All joints have a free blood supply with many anastomozing arteries. An operation on a major joint without a tourniquet provides a good demonstration of joint vascularity. There is a fine plexus of lymphatics within the synovial membranes.

The nerve supply of a joint is the same as that of the overlying muscles moving the joint and the skin over their insertions (Hilton's Law). Most of the nerve end-organs lie in the joint capsule, but muscle and tendon end-organs are equally important for proprioception. Autonomic nerves also reach the joint, mainly with the blood vessels, and control the blood supply and perhaps the formation of synovial fluid.

The protective and proprioceptive functions of nerves supplying joints are vital to the normal functioning of a joint, which rapidly disintegrates if this protection is lost (Charcot's joint).

Muscles

The functions of joints and muscles are closely interrelated. Not only are muscles important for moving the joints, but their co-ordinated action is essential for joint stability. This is very evident in paralytic conditions where the lack of stability may have to be compensated by the use of external splints.

Skeletal muscle is composed of fibres whose length varies from a few millimetres to about 30 cm. Each fibre contains many nuclei embedded in its syncytium and the fibre itself is built up of many myofibrils, each of which consists of units of the proteins actin and myosin. These are arranged in interlocking bands. They give the fibre its characteristic cross-sections, and are the contractile elements of the muscle.

The form of a muscle determines its power and contractility. If the fibres are arranged parallel to the line of pull, the contractility is greatest: where there are many fibres arranged obliquely to the line of pull, the power is greater but the ability to shorten is less.

Nerve supply to muscles

The nerve enters the muscle at the motor point, which is usually constant and is the point at which electrical stimulation is most effective. The smaller branches of each nerve fibre supply a variable number of muscle fibres, each junction being called a *motor end-plate*. Where fine control is needed, as with the small muscles of the hand, the number of muscle fibres supplied by each nerve fibre is small, whereas more coarsely innervated muscles may have one nerve fibre dividing to supply over a hundred motor end-plates. Afferent fibres derive from muscle spindles and are essential for the feedback mechanisms controlling contraction.

Muscles have many actions, sometimes functioning as prime movers, at other times as co-ordinating antagonists, synergists and co-operating muscles. Many of their so-called 'voluntary' activities are concerned with posture and are essentially unconscious.

Tendons and bursae

Most muscles are attached to the bone ends by a tendon, which may be a few millimetres or many centimetres long. Many of the larger tendons move within a fibrous sheath, which has a synovial lining (Fig. 1.6a).

Tendons do not resist pressure very well and are frequently separated or protected from their underlying bones by thin-walled cavities containing synovial fluid. Some of the larger tendons contain a bone within their substance at the place where they cross a joint and have to bear considerable stresses. These are known as *sesamoid bones*. Examples are the patella and the sesamoids under the first metatarsal head. They have articular cartilage on their deep surfaces (Fig. 1.6b).

Small sacs or *bursae* are often found overlying bony prominences. They may be fairly constant anatomical structures, like those overlying the

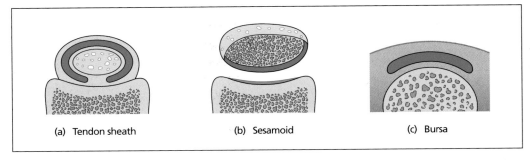

(a) Tendon sheath   (b) Sesamoid   (c) Bursa

Figure 1.6 Tendons and bursae. The darker blue areas indicate: (a) synovial sheath, (b) hyaline cartilage and (c) a fluid-filled bursa.

ischial tuberosity or olecranon, or they may be produced as a response to external pressure, when they are called 'adventitious' bursae, e.g. the one which develops over the patellar tendon in occupations involving continuous kneeling, or the first metatarsal head from pressure on the shoe (Fig. 1.6c). Certain anatomical bursae communicate with the nearby joint and may become distended or diseased if pathology develops in the underlying joint (such as a Baker's cyst).

Chapter 2

Soft-tissue injuries and healing

The term *soft tissues* refers to those parts which are not bone or cartilage. From the point of view of injuries, it is necessary to consider the skin, muscles, tendons, ligaments, blood vessels and nerves (the latter are discussed in Chapter 3). It is vital to consider not only what structures have been damaged, but also how the damage has come about, known as the *mechanism of injury*.

Mechanism of injury

Injuries may be either blunt or penetrating. They may occur by external insult, such as a cut by a knife, or indirectly, such as a nerve damaged by the sharp end of a bone. The amount of energy imparted to the soft tissues is proportional to the degree of violence applied.

Wound healing

Before discussing particular injuries, it is useful to consider how tissues heal. Many tissues do not regenerate when damaged and are repaired by collagenous scar tissue. Some tissues, such as bone, mucous membrane, liver and the superficial layers of skin, are capable of complete repair.

Lecture Notes: Orthopaedics and Fractures, 4e.
By T Duckworth and CM Blundell. Published 2010 by Blackwell Publishing.

Wound healing processes

The basic processes are seen best in the healing of a clean incised wound:

1 The wound bleeds and fills with clot

2 The inflammatory process is initiated and there is dilatation of capillaries, exudation of fluid and white cells, and the process of capillary budding begins

3 Dead tissue and clot are removed by phagocytes, and capillaries and fibroblasts migrate into the damaged area. The new tissue is known as *granulation tissue* and is highly vascular (2–3 days)

4 The skin surface begins to heal by the proliferation and migration of epithelial cells from the edges of the wound to cover the defect

5 The cellular reaction diminishes and the fibroblasts start to lay down collagen fibres (third day onwards)

6 Vascularity diminishes and the collagen increases

7 Scar contraction makes the defect much smaller. This effect is more marked in some areas than others, e.g. in the midline of the body, particularly over the back (2 weeks onwards)

8 Scar consolidation and further shrinkage occurs, and the scar becomes almost avascular.

The tensile strength of a wound increases to a safe functional level in 15 days and is back to normal in about 3 months, depending on the tissue.

Closure of wounds

With all wounds, particularly those communicating with a fracture or a joint, a decision has to be made as soon as possible about closure. This decision will normally depend on the degree of contamination of the wound, the extent of surrounding soft-tissue damage, the condition of the surrounding skin and the time which has elapsed since the injury. The decision may be altered by the circumstances of follow-up. Where the patient can be kept under observation, primary wound closure may be attempted in circumstances which might be considered too risky if close follow-up were not possible as, for example, in wartime conditions. If the decision has been made to close the wound, this should be done as soon as possible. Closure is best achieved with skin, either by direct suture or, for larger defects, by skin grafting.

1 **Primary closure** is usually safe if carried out in the first 6 hours after injury, provided all foreign material and dead tissue is removed, there is no communication with a fracture and there is little surrounding soft-tissue damage. A clean incised wound may be safely sutured up to 8 hours after injury. After this time, contamination is almost unavoidable and the risk of infection is much greater. It is then usually safer to leave the wound open and, after 24 hours, if it remains clean, perform:

2 **Delayed primary closure.**

3 **Secondary closure**, which means closure after the wound has been allowed to granulate, having overcome any sepsis. This may be at 4–5 days or up to several weeks after the injury. Suture may still be possible at this late stage, but frequently, skin grafting will be necessary. Large defects fill initially with granulation tissue, which is very resistant to infection. An area of clean granulation tissue is the best bed for a skin graft when primary grafting is not possible. Grafting in the presence of severe infection is usually unsuccessful, and tendons, ligaments and, particularly, articular cartilage, do not usually form suitable beds for non-vascularized grafts.

Following burns, areas of skin slough may need to be excised when demarcation has occurred, and the defect may then be covered by a suitable graft.

Techniques of closure

Suture

Suture materials may be absorbable or non-absorbable. Sutures are either deep or superficial and may be put in as a continuous stitch or as interrupted individual stitches. Skin may alternatively be apposed by adhesive dressings (e.g. butterfly sutures).

Skin grafting

1 **Partial thickness or split-skin grafting.** This is the easiest and most reliable technique and uses split skin taken from a convenient donor site. It may be used as a primary or secondary technique. It utilizes only part of the thickness of the epidermis and, if it is correctly taken, the donor site should bleed from the skin papillae only and will re-epithelialize spontaneously.

The graft may be held in place with dressings or suture. 'Superglue' has also been used with success to hold grafts in place during healing.

2 **Full-thickness detached grafts.** Until recently these have been rarely used except for small areas, such as defects on the fingers. When used as free grafts, they are much less likely than split skin to 'take' adequately. With the development of techniques for microvascular anastomosis, there is now much more interest in using various types of 'free' full-thickness grafts, either of skin alone or using thicker grafts of skin, subcutaneous tissue and muscle. It is also possible, for special requirements, to transfer composite grafts of skin, soft tissues and bone, a technique which is being increasingly used for the management of difficult open fractures, particularly of the tibia.

3 **Attached skin flaps.** These are the more conventional types of full-thickness grafts which may be rotated or swung, taken from one limb to another, or from chest or abdomen to limb. Considerable skill is needed to obtain good results. They provide much more satisfactory skin cover, but leave a defect elsewhere, which has to be closed by split skin. They resist pressure better and are essential for exposed and prominent areas. They

are usually detached from the donor site in 10–15 days and may require further adjustment later.

4 Foreign skin. Taken either from animal or human, this is occasionally used as a temporary dressing for large areas of loss, e.g. after burns. It is eventually rejected and secondary grafting may then be needed.

Types of wound

Superficial wounds

Abrasions

These are caused by trauma to the superficial skin layers, usually by friction. They heal with little scarring, but any foreign material should be removed by scrubbing or scraping; otherwise 'tattooing' will result.

Treatment
A simple protective dressing is usually all that is required.

Incised wounds

These are usually relatively uncontaminated and heal well with little scarring.

Lacerations

These may be clean and very similar to incised wounds, but are caused by blunt trauma and may be associated with crushing and haematoma formation in the surrounding tissues. Sometimes the skin can be sheared from the deeper layers, termed a *degloving injury*.

Treatment
All dead and foreign material should be excised and the wound closed by one of the methods described above. If there is any possibility of a foreign body, an X-ray is essential. Most foreign bodies, such as metal, stone or glass, are radio-opaque to some extent, but some materials, notably wood, are not visible on ordinary X-rays.

Burns

These may be partial thickness, that is within the epidermis, or full thickness—through the whole skin and into the subcutaneous or deeper tissues. The distinction is not always clear at the time of injury, but loss of sensation in the area is suggestive of full-thickness loss.

Treatment
Partial thickness burns usually heal rapidly and completely; if full thickness, the damaged tissue will slough and eventually separate or may need to be excised. The resulting wound is then closed by suture or more usually by skin grafting. Extensive burns are best dealt with in special units where facilities exist for the control of fluid loss, sepsis and later reconstruction.

Deep wounds

These may be extensions of lacerations or burns, or caused by a stabbing type of injury, when they may be much more widespread than is apparent from the surface.

Treatment
Any penetrating wound where there is the possibility of important soft-tissue damage should be explored. This is particularly important with stab wounds of the chest and abdomen, where extensive internal injury may be associated with a minor skin wound. In these circumstances, a laparotomy or thoracotomy may be necessary to achieve an adequate exploration.

Haematoma

This is a collection of blood in the tissues. If small, it will usually resolve and be replaced by scar tissue. If larger, it may fail to resolve completely, leaving a cyst which occasionally may expand and destroy surrounding tissues. This is particularly likely to happen in bleeding disorders such as haemophilia. Haematomas may become infected and lead to the development of an abscess.

Treatment

Large haematomata, particularly in confined spaces, may need decompression or evacuation to prevent necrosis of overlying tissues. Resorption may be speeded by active use of the limb. Secondary infection of a haematoma is not uncommon.

Contusion

This is the same as a bruise and consists of tissue damaged by a blow or crush. It is usually swollen and infiltrated with blood.

Foreign bodies

If sterile or non-irritative, these may cause little trouble, or may not be recognized. They frequently do cause a local reaction or abscess and may be the cause of a continually draining sinus.

Treatment

Removal is not always necessary, but if it is considered desirable, it should be carried out in good theatre conditions, with a tourniquet if possible, and with X-ray facilities available in case of difficulty.

Gunshot wounds

These are increasingly seen in civilian life as the use of firearms is becoming more commonplace. Missile injuries are usually classified as being of low-velocity or high-velocity types. In civilian practice the former are commoner since these are usually caused by revolvers or hand guns which deliver a heavy bullet at relatively low velocity— around 200 m/s. The bullets from rifles, such as the AK47 Assault rifle, travel at much higher velocities—up to 1000 m/s, or even higher. Though they may be smaller bullets, the energy released in the tissues, being derived from the high kinetic energy of the projectile, is much greater, causing more widespread and serious damage. The fragments thrown out of an exploding bomb or shell similarly behave as high-velocity missiles, causing correspondingly serious wounds.

Low-velocity gunshot wounds

The extent of this type of wound depends on how much the bullet is slowed and whether it is brought to rest in the tissues. This is influenced by the stability of the bullet. A stable perforating bullet may only release a small proportion of its available energy and cause relatively little damage.

In general, low-velocity wounds tend to be well circumscribed, with the tissues surrounding the track being damaged for a few millimetres only. The injury may not, therefore, be serious provided no important structure is directly hit.

Treatment

This consists essentially of excising foreign, necrotic and contaminated material. The extent of this excision may be quite small and the trend is to keep the surgery to a minimum. Fractures can usually be managed by standard techniques, wounds being left open with a view to secondary closure.

High-velocity gunshot wounds

Here, although the projectile and the entry wound may be small and innocent-looking, the amount of damage sustained by the internal tissues is often very extensive, due mainly to the phenomenon known as cavitation. This is caused by the violent acceleration of the tissues around the path of the missile, producing a large cavity which subsequently collapses, leaving necrotic tissue extending over a wide area around the track. During cavity formation, air and debris are sucked in through the entry wound so that in addition to widespread necrosis there may be much contamination. These effects may be particularly severe in the case of wounds of the chest, abdomen and head, causing widespread and often fatal damage. Fractures can be very severe with gross comminution.

Treatment

The management of this type of wound can present many surgical problems but, in principle, wounds should be opened widely, and extensive debridement and decompression carried out. All foreign and non-viable tissue must be removed and the wound left open. Wounds of the abdomen and chest will normally require exploration, and tissues such as bowel and liver can be expected to be much more severely damaged than they appear at first sight.

Injuries to organs

These are common, often occurring with blunt trauma such as in road traffic accidents. They are not always easy to recognize as they are not necessarily associated with superficial damage. Particularly vulnerable are the lungs, liver, spleen and genitourinary tract. Cerebral damage often follows head injury, whether the skull is fractured or not.

Injuries to ligaments

Joint injuries frequently involve complete rupture or partial tearing of ligaments. The latter is usually called a *sprain* or *strain*. Commonly injured are the ligaments of the knee and ankle (Fig. 2.1). Adequate diagnosis requires careful clinical assessment.

Occasionally stress X-rays are used to confirm the diagnosis.

Treatment

Sprains or partial tears usually heal with minimal treatment. They are usually painful in the acute stage and respond to immobilization with Elastoplast strapping or, in more severe cases, a plaster-cast. During the first 24 hours the symptoms can be helped by the use of ice or cold water compresses applied repeatedly, evaporation from the surface helping to maintain the cooling effect. As the pain settles the joint should be mobilized to avoid stiffness. Physiotherapy may be required. Recovery is usual in 2–3 weeks.

A complete ligament rupture requires apposition of the divided ends followed by a period of protection if satisfactory healing is to be obtained. Depending on the situation, the injury may be treated conservatively by immobilization in a plaster-cast or, preferably, in a functional brace designed to allow joint movement whilst restricting the stresses on the healing ligament. If there is reason to doubt whether the torn ends are in apposition, surgical suture may be advisable. Three weeks' protection is usually sufficient to secure

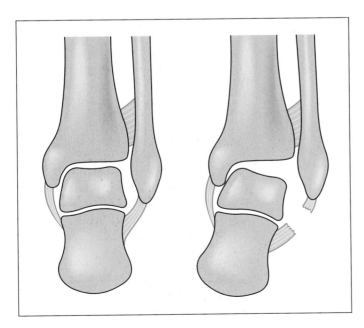

Figure 2.1 Diagram to show ligament rupture.

healing and mobilization can then be gradually increased.

The widespread use of pain-relieving injections into the damaged ligaments of athletes and sportsmen is to be deplored, since further damage can occur without the patient being aware of it.

Injuries to tendons

Tendons are frequently divided by injury. When the injury is recognized, suture may be possible at the time the wound is closed. This is usually done with a wire mono-filament Kessler's suture and protecting the repair by splintage for a period of 3–6 weeks (Fig. 2.2).

In the case of the finger flexor tendons in the zone between the distal palmar crease and the proximal interphalangeal joint—usually called 'no-man's land' (Fig. 2.3)—primary suture of both tendons is indicated whenever possible, but in this area the tendons run within the flexor tendon sheaths and skill is required to achieve good results because of the tendency for adhesions to form in the sheath. In less skilled hands, it is safer to close the skin and perform a tendon repair or grafting operation later. Protected movement by careful splintage is an important part of the overall treatment. The 'Belfast' regime, which involves splinting the finger in partial flexion but allowing some degree of active flexion, has become popular in the UK as it reduces adhesion formation.

Traditionally, if both flexor tendons were divided in 'no man's land', only flexor digitorum profundus (FDP) was repaired and flexor digitorum superficialis (FDS) was left, but increasingly with regimes allowing greater early movement, both

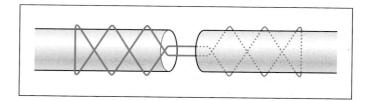

Figure 2.2 Tendon suture.

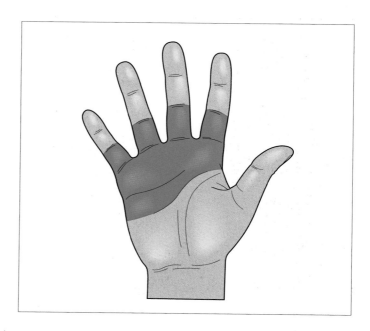

Figure 2.3 No-man's land.

tendons are repaired directly if possible. If there is loss of tendon length after debridement, a tendon graft using palmaris longus or a toe extensor may be used. Sometimes a silastic 'former' is placed in the finger to form a track or tunnel prior to the insertion of the tendon graft. The finger must be mobile before the grafting procedure and vigorous physiotherapy is usually necessary afterwards.

Injuries to vessels

Any injured limb should be examined for evidence of ischaemia. Excessive swelling, especially if it is increasing, should arouse suspicion, and failure to secure return of circulation when a fracture is reduced should be an indication for exploration and, if necessary, repair of vessels. Commonly injured are the femoral artery and the arteries of the lower leg. The aorta is occasionally ruptured in multiple injuries and this may be difficult to differentiate from other causes of shock. Occasionally, if a damaged vessel has not been repaired or ligated, a false aneurysm may develop at the point of rupture and this may expand or possibly rupture in its turn, causing delayed ischaemic or pressure effects.

Treatment

If time allows, it is usual to assess the situation before surgery by angiography. With major vessels, suture may be possible or the vessel may have to be repaired with a vein patch or a graft, usually taken from a vein. Fasciotomy is usually necessary (see below).

Compartment syndromes

Occasionally, following trauma to a limb, particularly a closed fracture or crush injury, the venous outflow from a fascial compartment may become obstructed by swelling, causing the pressure to rise gradually within the compartment. When the pressure reaches a critical level, any nerves passing through the compartment cease to function, initially causing paraesthesiae, followed by loss of sensation in the area supplied by the nerve. As the pressure continues to rise, tissue perfusion may cease, particularly in the muscles, and, rarely, a

point may be reached when the pressure rises above arterial level and all structures within the compartment become ischaemic. If the pressure is not relieved urgently, the necrotic muscle may lead to the need for limb amputation. In less dramatic cases, the eventual replacement of the muscle by fibrous tissue may result in contracture of the muscle and deformity of the associated joints (*Volkmann's ischaemic contracture*).

Clinical features

The condition occurs most commonly following closed fractures of the tibia and fibula, but can arise in any of the fascial compartments of the upper or lower limbs and may follow open fractures or more proximal vascular injuries. The syndrome usually develops during the 24–48 hours after injury, but occasionally later. Pain at the site of the affected compartment is usually the earliest and most important feature, with paraesthesiae, numbness and muscular weakness developing later. The pain is typically made worse by stretching the affected muscles, which are also tender. Swelling of the ankle, foot or hand is not necessarily a feature. Neurological signs eventually develop if the pressure is not released and in the late case the peripheral pulses may become impalpable. Presence or absence of the pulses is *not*, however, a good guide to the diagnosis.

Treatment

The most important aspect of management is an awareness that the condition may develop. If any of the above features appear, the condition should be suspected. It is possible to measure the intra-compartmental pressures using a simple manometric device and pressures within 30 mmHg of the diastolic blood pressure are usually regarded as an indication for decompression. This is carried out by splitting the deep fascia over the length of the compartment (*fasciotomy*). The skin is also often left open. In the lower leg it may be necessary to decompress all four muscle compartments. If the equipment is not available for measuring the pressures, decompression should be carried out on clinical suspicion. At the time of debridement all necrotic tissue must be removed.

Pressure sores

These arise from continued pressure, usually over a bony prominence. They are essentially ischaemic and more likely to occur if there is loss of sensation. They are preventable by avoiding long periods of continuous pressure. Three to 4 hours may be sufficient to cause skin necrosis. The sacrum and heels are the most vulnerable sites for true bed sores and these can usually be avoided by moving or turning the patient every 2 hours. Pressure sores from splints and plasters are also common.

Treatment

It is better to go to considerable trouble to prevent pressure sores than to have to treat them, because they are difficult to heal. Small sores will often heal with simple dressings, after removal of sloughs if necessary. The most important factor in successful treatment is to avoid further pressure. Large sores may require wide surgical excision and skin grafting, often by the rotation of thick flaps of skin and subcutaneous tissue. Chronic peripheral ulcers, caused by pressure and usually associated with sensory loss, can often be healed by enclosing the limb in a series of 'skin-tight' plaster-casts and avoiding weight-bearing until healing has occurred.

Self-inflicted injuries

Any recurrent haematoma or recurrent bleeding which is apparently inexplicable should arouse suspicion of self-infliction. The dorsum of the hand and wrist is a particularly common site. A period in a plaster-cast will usually allow healing, but the damage may recur when the plaster is removed. These injuries often cease when their cause has been discovered.

Chapter 3

Nerve injuries and repair

Peripheral nerve injuries

The importance of these merits their separate discussion. Peripheral nerve injuries may be caused by one of the following:

1 Direct trauma, e.g. lacerations, gunshot wounds, penetrating injuries, burns, etc

2 Indirect trauma, e.g. fracture fragments may stretch or tear a nerve. A fracture may also produce delayed effects on a nerve. A good example is the palsy caused by the ulnar nerve being stretched around the medial side of an elbow which has grown into valgus as a result of damage to the lateral epicondylar epiphysis (Fig. 3.1)

3 Chronic or acute entrapment, e.g. the median nerve may be trapped within the carpal tunnel as a result of fracture, or disease of the wrist or tendon sheaths—as seen, for example, in rheumatoid arthritis. There are a number of such 'tunnel syndromes', often with no obvious cause, but producing characteristic clinical pictures.

Carpal tunnel syndrome

This condition tends to occur in young to middle-aged women and is particularly likely to occur

Lecture Notes: Orthopaedics and Fractures, 4e.
By T Duckworth and CM Blundell. Published 2010 by Blackwell Publishing.

during pregnancy. It is occasionally an early manifestation of rheumatoid arthritis.

Clinical features

The presenting symptom is usually pain or paraesthesiae in the thumb, index and middle fingers, often occurring at night and sometimes relieved by hanging the arm out of bed. Some patients complain of numbness or clumsiness when carrying out fine manipulations.

There may be obvious wasting of the thenar muscles, lack of sweating over the median nerve distribution and occasionally objective sensory loss. Pressure over the carpal tunnel may reproduce the symptoms. Nerve conduction studies may be needed to confirm the diagnosis.

Treatment

Those cases developing during pregnancy often settle after delivery. A trial of a plaster back-slab to immobilize the wrist is often useful. An injection of a steroid preparation into the carpal tunnel is often helpful, but persistent cases can be relieved quickly by operative decompression of the carpal tunnel, although muscle wasting may be permanent.

Acute peripheral nerve injuries

Nerves may be injured at the root, plexus or trunk level, and severe injuries to the major plexuses may result in avulsion of the roots from the spinal cord.

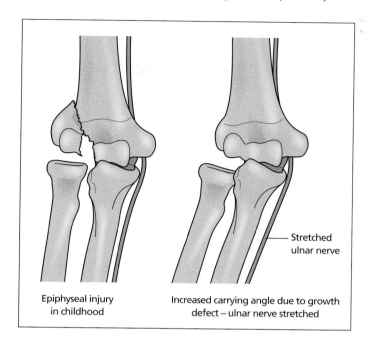

Epiphyseal injury
in childhood

Increased carrying angle due to growth
defect – ulnar nerve stretched

Stretched
ulnar nerve

Figure 3.1 Delayed ulnar nerve palsy due to fracture.

Diagnosis

Nerve injuries can usually be accurately diagnosed by a careful consideration of the detailed neurological anatomy. A systematic examination should be carried out, recording the power of all muscle groups, the distribution of sensory loss to various modalities, and the presence or absence of reflexes. In the difficult case, electromyography or conduction studies and occasionally myelography may help to clarify the diagnosis and the prognosis. These tests are also valuable in following the progress of denervation and recovery.

Recovery from trauma

Peripheral nerves are capable of repair after injury. Three types of damage are theoretically possible:

1 Neurapraxia. This is usually due to blunt trauma or compression. The axons remain in continuity and usually recover quickly over minutes, hours or occasionally longer. The condition is analogous to cerebral concussion.

2 Axonotmesis. This involves damage to individual axons but within intact sheaths. It may be caused by direct trauma or by stretching. In the latter case the prognosis is usually worse. Axons regenerate from the central end, provided the cell body remains alive, and recovery should be good if the fibres are able to grow down their original neurilemmal sheaths. Recovery depends on axons reaching appropriate end-organs and may take months in the case of the longer nerves, such as the sciatic.

3 Neuronotmesis. In this condition the nerve is completely divided or irreparably damaged over part of its length. Each divided axon tends to die back to the next node of Ranvier or even further, and there are usually retrograde changes in the motor cell body. The peripheral axon disintegrates, the myelin sheath breaks up and the neurilemmal cells become disorganized. Recovery follows in the same way as after axonotmesis, but the reconnections of fibres and end-organs are likely to be much less satisfactory. Regeneration rarely occurs unless the nerve ends are opposed. At best, recovery tends to be incomplete, although the prognosis is much better in children. Clean divisions, with little trauma on either side of the lesion, have the best prognosis, and the more peripheral the lesion, the better the outlook.

Nerve repair

Primary suture

This is possible with clean wounds and cleanly divided nerves. It is usually necessary to cut back the nerve ends to remove nerve tissue damaged by bleeding within the sheath. If much cutting back or excision of a length has been necessary, the nerve will have to be mobilized up and down the limb and perhaps the joints flexed to allow apposition. On occasions the nerve ends are glued together. Suture is carried out using very fine sutures passed through the nerve sheath. Modern techniques involve suturing individual nerve bundles, under microscopic vision. If primary repair is not thought possible, the ends should be loosely labelled with a suture and tacked together, and the wound then closed.

Secondary suture

This can be carried out when the skin wound is healed and up to 6 months after the injury. The scarred and thickened junction is excised and again the nerve is mobilized and the sheath sutured. Secondary suture may require more excision of the nerve, but operative conditions and expertise may be more favourable. After both methods of suture the repair is protected by immobilizing the joints for several weeks. If the gap is too great for suturing, grafting is possible, using a sensory nerve such as the sural which can be sacrificed without too much functional loss. Nerve grafts can be bundled together to allow several strips of small nerve to function as a larger nerve. Results tend to be indifferent. An interesting experimental technique involves the use of strips of muscle as a nerve graft.

Tinel's sign

This is a useful sign for following recovery. Gentle tapping with the fingertip along the course of the nerve will result in the patient feeling pins and needles in the distribution of the nerve when the point of regeneration is reached. This point will gradually move more distally as recovery proceeds.

Brachial plexus injuries

These produce complex neurological pictures. Some common patterns can be discerned.

Birth injuries

These are now rare and usually occur as a result of traction or pressure during delivery.

They have a variable prognosis. Some recovery occurs in at least 50% of cases of Erb's palsy, the commonest type, affecting the upper plexus, but the lower plexus injuries carry a worse prognosis.

Other and mixed patterns

These are fairly common following road accidents, especially motorcycling, where the neck may be violently flexed laterally and the shoulder depressed.

Plexus injuries, in general, have a poor prognosis, particularly if the injury is proximal to the dorsal root ganglia. This is an important prognostic point. With injuries to the higher roots the exact site of damage may be obscure, but if the injury is proximal, myelography or MRI scanning may reveal the damage to the root sleeves. If the first thoracic root is injured proximally to its ganglion, Horner's syndrome will be present because the sympathetic outflow from the spinal cord passes through this root. Horner's syndrome is characterized by pupillary constriction, enophthalmos and ptosis, with some degree of loss of sweating on the affected side of the face.

Treatment

For birth palsies, this consists simply of maintaining passive joint movements by physiotherapy, in anticipation of recovery.

Attempts at reconstruction of the plexus following most types of injury are rarely successful, although better results are claimed for early exploration and suture performed in specialist centres. Some recovery may occur over the first 1 or even 2 years following a severe brachial plexus injury. When this has reached its maximum, reconstructive procedures on the arm may be considered. Unfortunately, chronic pain is often a disabling feature and may prevent satisfactory rehabilitation. Severe plexus injuries may eventually require amputation of the limb because of persistent pain, but unfortunately, even this drastic step does not always succeed in relieving the pain.

Injuries to nerve trunks

Median nerve

This is most commonly damaged at the wrist, occasionally in the forearm, or at the elbow. The neurological loss is mainly sensory, producing anaesthesia over the thumb, index, middle and, occasionally, ring fingers. Its effects on hand function are considerable. Lesions at wrist level produce paralysis and wasting of the thenar muscles, with the exception of the adductor pollicis, which is supplied by the ulnar nerve. Higher lesions may paralyse the flexor digitorum profundus to the index and middle fingers, and usually the whole of flexor digitorum superficialis, so that the index finger cannot be actively flexed at either interphalangeal joint.

Ulnar nerve

The loss here is mainly motor. Damage may occur at any level, but it is commonest at the wrist or elbow. The intrinsic muscles in the hand, when working normally, put the fingers into a position of flexion at the metacarpophalangeal joints and extension at the interphalangeal joints. When these muscles are paralysed by an ulnar nerve lesion, the fingers take up the opposite position ('clawing') due to the unopposed long flexors (Fig. 3.2). This effect is less in the index because the first two lumbricals are innervated by the median nerve. Thumb adduction is lost (but may be disguised). The long flexors to the ring and little fingers and the ulnar wrist flexors may be lost in high lesions, in which case clawing does not occur, known as the 'ulnar nerve paradox'. Sensation is lost over the little and part of the ring fingers.

Radial nerve

This is usually damaged at the level of the mid-humerus by fractures or pressure, e.g. going to sleep with the arm over the back of a chair, known as 'Saturday night palsy'. The lesion results in paralysis of wrist, finger and thumb extensors, and a characteristic 'drop wrist'. The motor branch to the triceps is often spared. There is usually little sensory loss.

Sciatic nerve

This is occasionally damaged in association with a dislocated hip. Division of the sciatic nerve is a serious injury producing complete loss of function and almost total anaesthesia below the knee (with the exception of the saphenous nerve, which arises from the femoral nerve).

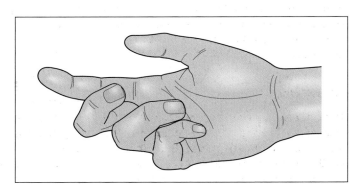

Figure 3.2 Claw hand after ulnar nerve palsy.

Femoral nerve

Femoral nerve palsy is often caused by penetrating injuries, e.g. by a butcher's knife. Its main effect is loss of quadriceps function, making standing and walking difficult. Stairs are particularly difficult to manage. The patient may learn to brace his knee back by using his hand, producing a very characteristic gait.

Common peroneal nerve

This is commonly injured, often following splintage, because the nerve is vulnerable where it winds round the neck of the fibula. Its loss produces a drop foot with anaesthesia over the dorsum. This often fails to recover and a toe-raising appliance may eventually be needed to correct the tendency to catch the toe when walking (see p. 231, Fig. 24.11).

Time of recovery

Axons are capable of regenerating at the rate of 1 mm/day. It is, therefore, possible to calculate roughly how long will be necessary before functional recovery can be expected.

Chapter 4

Fractures and healing

Fractures

A fracture is a break in continuity of a bone. A *comminuted* fracture is one with more than two fragments. Gross comminution is usually caused by severe violence and in such cases union is often delayed or difficult to achieve.

Describing fractures

The type of fracture which occurs depends on the magnitude and direction of the force causing it.

1 **Transverse fracture.** This is usually caused by a force applied directly to the site at which the fracture occurs. This often represents a three-point force system (Fig. 4.1).

2 **Spiral or oblique fracture.** This is produced by a twisting force applied distant from the site of the fracture, usually at each end of a long bone such as the tibia (Fig. 4.2).

3 **Greenstick fracture.** This occurs in children, whose bones are soft and yielding. The bone bends without fracturing across completely, the cortex on the concave side usually remaining intact (Fig. 4.3).

4 **Crush fracture.** This occurs in cancellous bone as a result of a compression force (Fig. 4.4).

5 **Burst fracture.** This usually occurs in a short bone, such as a vertebra from strong direct pressure; in the vertebrae this usually occurs as a result of impaction of the disc (Fig. 4.5).

6 **Avulsion fracture.** This is caused by traction, a bony fragment usually being torn off by a tendon or ligament (Fig. 4.6).

7 **Fracture dislocation or subluxation.** This is a fracture which involves a joint and results in malalignment of the joint surfaces (Figs 4.7 and 4.8).

A surface wound may communicate with a fracture. This is known as an *open* fracture. An open fracture sometimes communicates with an internal body surface, e.g. a pelvic fracture may communicate with a rupture of the rectum or a rib fracture may penetrate a lung. Open fractures are potentially infected and need urgent treatment.

All fractures involve some soft-tissue damage, but when there is important soft-tissue damage to nerves, vessels or internal organs, then the fracture is termed *complicated*. Occasionally, the bone ends may be separated by soft tissue, such as muscle, and this may delay union.

A fracture is *impacted* when the fragments are driven into one another. Such a fracture is usually *stable*, as also is a fracture which is held firmly by soft-tissue attachments, usually periosteum. An *unstable* fracture is one which is displaced or has the potential to displace. Occasionally, when a fracture is realigned or *reduced*, the fragments lock together and the fracture then becomes stable.

Lecture Notes: Orthopaedics and Fractures, 4e.
By T Duckworth and CM Blundell. Published 2010 by Blackwell Publishing.

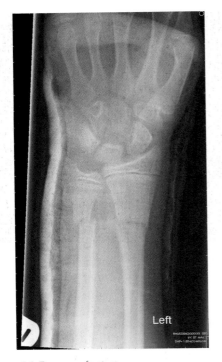

Figure 4.1 Transverse fracture.

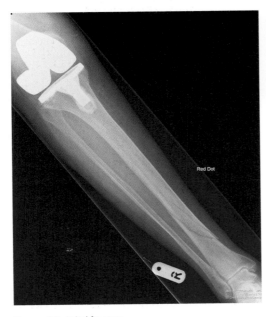

Figure 4.2 Spiral fracture.

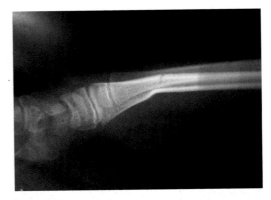

Figure 4.3 Greenstick fracture.

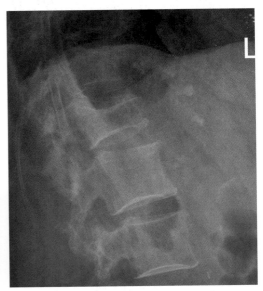

Figure 4.4 Crush fracture.

More usually, following reduction, the fracture will re-displace if not held in some way. If the periosteum is intact on one side, this may be used to help secure stability.

Displacement may mean shortening, rotation, sideways shift or tilt, and reduction of the fracture will usually involve reversing these various displacements.

A *dislocation* is a complete loss of congruity of the joint surfaces. A *subluxation* is a partial loss of contact of the joint surfaces. Either may be associ-

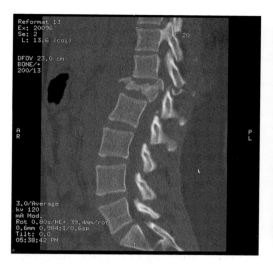

Figure 4.5 Burst fracture.

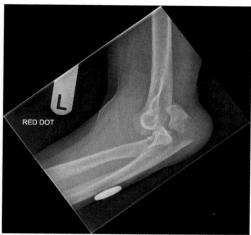

Figure 4.7 Fracture dislocation.

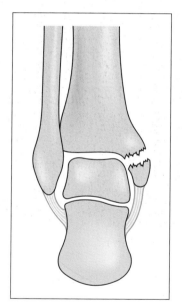

Figure 4.6 Avulsion fracture.

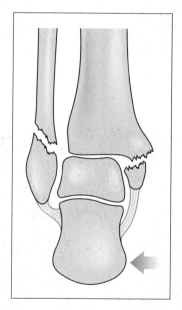

Figure 4.8 Fracture subluxation.

ated with a fracture and may, of course, be an open injury.

An *intra-articular* fracture is one in which the fracture involves the joint surface. Usually these fractures require operative anatomical reduction if there is displacement.

Epiphyseal injuries occur in children. In certain circumstances they may interfere with growth. The Salter and Harris classification is usually used for these injuries (Table 4.1 and Fig. 4.9). The fracture line normally runs through the calcifying layer of the epiphysis on the side away from the germinal

Table 4.1 Salter and Harris classification.

Type I	The fracture line passes cleanly along the epiphyseal line with no metaphyseal fragment. This type tends to occur in young children or babies and in pathological conditions such as spina bifida or scurvy
Type II	The commonest type, in which the fracture line runs across the epiphyseal line and then obliquely, shearing off a small triangle of metaphysis
Type III	The epiphysis may be split vertically and a fragment displaced along the epiphyseal line
Type IV	The fracture extends through the epiphyseal line from the metaphysis into the epiphysis. This type may interfere with growth because union may take place across the growth plate
Type V	Severe crushing of the epiphysis may occur from longitudinal compression and this is very likely to result in growth arrest and deformity

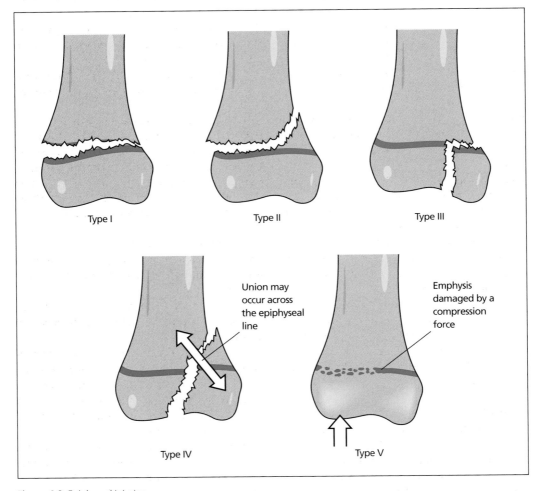

Figure 4.9 Epiphyseal injuries.

layer. The first three types have a good prognosis and are usually easy to reduce, provided they are treated early by manipulation. The third type tends to occur in older children and adolescents and, since it is intra-articular, may require open reduction and pinning in position.

Diagnosing fractures

Many fractures can be readily diagnosed from the history or from the fact that the limb is malaligned.

History

A brief history is essential in order to assess the mechanism of injury and to raise suspicion of other, less apparent, injuries. If the violence has been minimal and hardly sufficient to have caused a fracture, then this may arouse a suspicion that the fractured bone has been weakened by disease or previous damage, a so-called *pathological* fracture.

1 **Pain.** This is the commonest symptom, but varies with the site and instability of the fracture. Individuals also vary greatly in their response to pain.

2 **Loss of function.** There is almost always some impairment of function in the injured area, so that the patient may be unable to move the limb at all, or may use it with difficulty. Some degree of function may be retained. Following a femoral neck fracture, for example, the patient may manage to walk, but always limps and there is always some functional impairment.

3 **Loss of sensation or motor power.** This is a particularly important symptom, suggesting nerve or vascular complications. The time of injury should be ascertained as accurately as possible, especially with an open fracture or where there are signs of ischaemia.

Physical signs

The classical signs of a fracture may or may not be present.

1 **Tenderness** is almost invariable with a recent fracture, assuming the patient is conscious. Its exact distribution should be determined.

2 **Deformity** may or may not be evident. The limb may be bent or shortened, or there may be a step in the alignment of the bone or joint.

3 **Swelling** is usual when the fracture is fairly superficial; gross swelling usually implies a vascular rupture. Swelling takes some time to appear and may increase over the first 12–24 hours. It is sometimes associated with blistering of the skin. Swelling is partly due to haematoma, partly due to inflammatory exudation. There may be obvious bruising. A joint which is fractured may fill with blood *haemarthrosis*.

4 **Local temperature increase** is essentially part of the inflammatory response which rapidly follows the injury and may be evident even if the damage is confined to the soft tissues.

5 **Abnormal mobility or crepitus**, i.e. grating of the fracture ends, may be noticed. Vigorous attempts to elicit it should be avoided.

6 **Loss of function** is almost always found to some extent. The patient usually has difficulty in moving the adjacent joints.

Having diagnosed a fracture or joint injury, the presence and extent of any wound should be noted, and the area examined for evidence of ischaemia and nerve or other important soft-tissue damage. This is essential routine in examining any injury of the musculoskeletal system. Other injuries should also be suspected and sought.

Radiological examination

The X-ray examination is designed to give information additional to that obtained by clinical judgement (Box 4.1).

X-rays in at least two planes, usually at right angles, are essential. A fracture may be missed if only one film is taken.

Some fractures may elude both clinical and radiological diagnosis, and treatment may have to rest on suspicion initially, with X-ray changes occurring later as bone resorption occurs, such as a scaphoid bone fracture, sometimes only seen on a radionuclide bone scan.

Computed tomography (CT) scanning has become a useful aid in diagnosing the more difficult injuries, particularly fractures of the pelvis, spine and complex intra-articular fractures. It can be useful for planning the details of surgery when open reduction is contemplated.

Fracture healing

This follows the same steps as soft-tissue wound healing, except that the migrating cells have osteogenic potential (i.e. can make bone), sometimes laying down cartilage as an intermediate stage (Fig. 4.10).

There is no general agreement about the source of the migrating cells. One theory is that they derive from specialized cells which are to be found on all free bone surfaces and particularly on the deep surface of the fibrous periosteum. These are

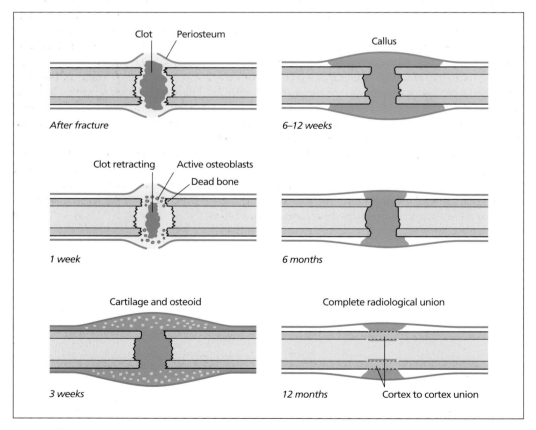

Figure 4.10 Fracture healing.

morphologically indistinguishable from fibroblasts but are thought to give rise to osteoblasts, which then lose the capacity to divide. The alternative theory is that the active cells are derived from non-specialized fibroblasts in the surrounding soft tissues and that these cells can develop the power to lay down bone, given the necessary stimulus. It has also been suggested that the osteogenic cells may be derived from marrow cells or even from vascular endothelium.

The ultimate aim of fracture healing may be considered to be what is called 'cortex-to-cortex' union, with bone directly joining the fracture surfaces, but this is essentially a slow process and requires the fracture to be immobilized in some way before it can occur. Many fractures are joined initially and rapidly by a cuff of provisional woven bone known as *callus*. This varies in amount and is greatest when the fracture is allowed to move.

Fracture healing may involve several interlinked processes contributing in varying degrees to the healing of any individual fracture. It has been suggested that in the first few days and weeks there is a primary callus response occurring as a fundamental reaction to bone injury. This response is thought to be short-lived and peters out if it fails to provide satisfactory bridging between the fragments. In that case, a second mechanism may come into play called 'bridging external callus', possibly derived from a process of bone induction in surrounding soft-tissue cells and very dependent on blood vessels from these tissues. If this succeeds in providing a bridge, then end-to-end union can occur,

with remodelling and the gradual replacement of dead bone. Whether or not temporary bone bridging is achieved, a third process of bone union may become important in the later stages. This has been called late medullary callus and appears to be responsible for the slow growth of new bone across the fracture gap, and even, given a sufficient degree of stability, across a fibrous tissue barrier. It is very dependent on the bone circulation and may be inhibited by intramedullary internal fixation.

If the fracture is rigidly fixed, virtually no callus is seen and direct union across the fracture gap may eventually occur without a callus stage. In these circumstances, the rigid fixation takes the place of the callus. Rigid internal fixation may suppress or even replace the first two processes of fracture healing, and may cause the final stage of cortex-to-cortex union to be long delayed, because the fixation device takes most of the stresses. Because of the potential for rigid fixation to delay union, many fixation devices allow some movement to occur at the fracture. These devices allow the limb to be normally aligned, to take weight without displacement at the fracture site (so-called 'load sharing' devices), but also allow preservation of the normal healing process. External fixators and to a lesser extent intramedullary nails follow these principles.

Clinical union of a long bone in an adult normally takes about 3–4 months. There is then a gradual process of remodelling to produce cancellous and cortical bone with normal trabecular orientation.

Chapter 5

Fractures—principles of management

Having diagnosed the fracture accurately and carried out any resuscitation which may have been necessary, the fracture itself must be managed. The anatomy must be restored as closely as possible, the reduction must then be held such that the injured part and the patient as a whole may be rehabilitated. This is summarized as:

1 Reduce
2 Maintain reduction
3 Rehabilitate.

Open fractures

The treatment of these fractures is an orthopaedic emergency. The most important consideration when dealing with an open fracture is to reduce the risks of infection. The development of chronic osteomyelitis at the fracture site is a catastrophe, which may lead to delayed or non-union, requiring months or even years of treatment and sometimes leading to loss of the limb. There is general agreement that sepsis is best prevented by early and aggressive cleaning of the wound with excision of dead tissue and all foreign material. In order to achieve this, the wound often needs to be extended. Loose fragments of bone are devitalized and so should be removed, as should bone deep to

Lecture Notes: Orthopaedics and Fractures, 4e.
By T Duckworth and CM Blundell. Published 2010 by Blackwell Publishing.

areas where the periosteum has been stripped. This process of cleaning and removing devitalized tissue is termed *debridement.*

It is generally accepted that primary closure of wounds carries too much risk of deep sepsis and that all communicating wounds should be left open and covered with a sterile dressing, with a view to later closure when infection has been avoided or overcome. However, on occasions primary closure is desirable if it can be achieved safely, and some would advocate closure if the degree of contamination and soft-tissue damage is minimal and if the time from the accident is not too great, usually less than 6 hours. To this must be added the proviso that the patient should be kept under observation, preferably in hospital. If this philosophy is followed, then each case is judged on its merits. Generally, leaving the wound for secondary closure or skin cover is safer. *Antibiotics* should always be given after culture swabs have been taken. There is general agreement that in wartime conditions, where transportation may be necessary, communicating wounds are better left open. If primary closure is not considered appropriate, every attempt should be made to close the wound within 72 hours.

Open fractures are emergencies

Closure is usually achieved by one of the methods of skin grafting, remembering that bone cannot be covered directly by split-skin grafting, and if exposed a soft-tissue flap will be needed (see Chapter 2). The precise method of closure may depend on the method of treating the fracture itself, so these decisions must be made together. It is good practice to involve plastic surgeons early in the management of open fractures.

Reduction

Does the fracture need reduction?

Fractures do not always need reduction, but if the following apply then they do for several reasons.

1 Function. If the fracture is left to unite in the displaced position, often there will be functional impairment, such as a short limb. In general, fractures involving joints require anatomical reduction if possible, because of the need for the surfaces to glide accurately. With fractures of the shafts of the radius and ulna, any malalignment is likely to cause restriction of pronation and supination; this may be considered to function like an intra-articular fracture. Limbs need to be well aligned, because if they are not there are risks of later joint degeneration due to abnormal loading at joints.

2 Mobility. For some fractures, in elderly patients particularly, prolonged immobility in traction, for example, is dangerous, and reduction with stability of the fracture allows early mobilization.

3 Union. Some fractures unite with difficulty, usually because of impaired blood supply. In these cases union may be helped by accurate reduction, which should give any remaining blood vessels a chance to function. A subcapital fracture of the femur is a good example.

4 Neurovascular compromise. There may be impacted soft tissues, especially nerves or blood vessels, which are being distorted by the fracture or trapped between the bone ends, and these may need to be extracted by reducing the fracture.

5 Cosmesis. The appearance of the limb may be unsatisfactory even though function may be reasonable, e.g. a fracture through the tibia may function perfectly well if left overlapping, but might look unsightly.

If none of these criteria applies, then the fracture may be left to unite in the displaced position.

Techniques of reduction

1 Manipulation under anaesthesia. This is the method adopted for most fractures and dislocations.

2 Traction. Some fractures and dislocations may be reduced slowly by traction. This is usually used when manipulation is inappropriate, perhaps because an anaesthetic would be dangerous, e.g. subluxation or dislocation of one or more facets of the cervical spine.

3 Open reduction. This has the advantage of allowing very accurate reduction, but carries the risk of infection. Usually, open reduction is reserved for those cases where closed methods will not give the desired reduction, or where internal fixation is going to be needed for some other reason (see below). Open reduction does not necessarily imply internal fixation, although usually it does.

4 Closed reduction and fixation. For some fractures, such as those treated by intramedullary nailing or by external fixation, the reduction is indirectly achieved, with traction and the fracture stabilized with a nail or a fixator.

Maintaining fracture reduction

Stability is achieved by one of the following techniques:

1 Intrinsic stability. Some fractures require no additional stabilization

2 External splintage.

3 Internal fixation.

External splintage

Before deciding which method of external splintage to use, it must be decided how accurately the fracture needs to be held. Many fractures can be adequately immobilized with a simple device, such as a splint made of wire, metal or polythene, bandaged in place, and a sling or crutches may be used to avoid load-bearing. These devices are often used to relieve pain rather than to secure immobilization.

Casting

Plaster of Paris is still widely used for making open or closed casts, jointed casts, splints, etc (Box. 5.1). Other types of moulded splint, e.g. polythene, plastazote, etc, are usually less convenient to make and fit, although they may have other advantages.

Because of the heaviness and ease of water damage, newer casting materials have been developed. Most of these are made from a fabric base impregnated with a resin which undergoes a setting process when activated by heat or water. They all have slightly different characteristics, but, in general, they have advantages over plaster of Paris in that they are light in weight, but very strong (Box 5.2). This means that the patient may be able to bear weight on an unprotected cast, and nursing and moving a patient with a larger cast may be simplified. Most of the newer materials are waterproof, but to make full use of this property, lining and padding materials also need to be waterproof or, at least, quick drying. The main disadvantages of these new materials are that they cannot be readily molded and are more expensive. Nonetheless, they are becoming widely adopted.

Box 5.1 Plaster of Paris—advantages.

- Cheap and easily available
- Versatile and readily applied and fashioned
- Reasonably comfortable
- Absorbs secretions to some extent
- Fairly strong
- Radio-translucent

Box 5.2 Plaster of Paris—disadvantages.

- Heavy and warm
- Unyielding, so may cause pressure problems, or uncertain immobilization
- Difficult to inspect the limb, so it may conceal trouble, e.g. wound breakdown or sepsis
- Not waterproof

Cast bracing

A cast brace is a hinged or jointed cast. This technique is popular, especially with light-weight materials. It has been used particularly for fractures of the femur and tibia, although the principle is now being extended to the treatment of other fractures. The cast is accurately moulded around the limb using some of the techniques developed by limb fitters, and specially designed hinges are used to connect the various segments. The femoral cast brace has the advantages of allowing the joints to be exercised and the patient to be mobilized, whilst avoiding the risks of internal fixation. If a cast brace is to be used, it is usual to treat a femoral shaft fracture by traction until it is considered to be stable, usually at about 3–6 weeks. The cast is then applied and the patient allowed to mobilize. Full weight-bearing is usually permitted and, indeed, encouraged. The device may be used both to secure reduction and then to hold the position. Its use has diminished with the increasing interest in internal fixation.

Traction

Traction is pulling bones directly or indirectly in order to reduce and hold fractures. Historically traction has been a mainstay of fracture treatment around the world. It is a technique used less often now with the increasing use of internal fixation. Where hospital inpatient costs are high, traction, which often necessitates the patient remaining in hospital, is used less.

Methods of applying traction

1 Skin traction. The force is exerted tangentially along the skin by using adhesive strapping to attach the cord and weight. This is satisfactory for many purposes, but the force which can be applied is limited by the damage it may cause to the skin over time. Many people become sensitive to the adhesive.

2 Skeletal traction. This is applied by means of a pin or similar device applied directly through bone (Fig. 5.1). It enables greater force to be used, but may allow infection into the bone.

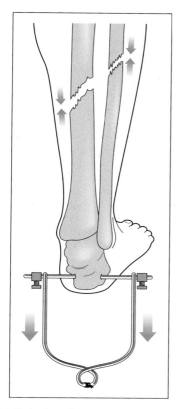

Figure 5.1 Skeletal traction.

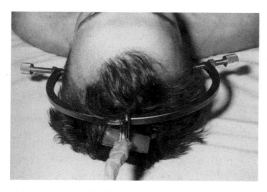

Figure 5.2 Gardner–Wells skull calipers.

Traction may be applied to the skull by means of tongs inserted into the calvarium (Fig. 5.2).

Fixed traction

The traction is applied against a counter force applied to the patient's body, e.g. a collar and cuff sling utilizes the weight of the arm to apply traction to the upper arm or shoulder. The counter force is applied to the part of the sling which passes around the patient's neck. The Thomas' splint is the best example of fixed traction using an orthopaedic appliance, the counter force being applied to the ischial tuberosity (and the overlying skin and soft tissues) (Fig. 5.3).

Sliding or balanced traction

The patient's weight is balanced against an applied load, utilizing frictional and gravitational forces to counterbalance the applied traction. Sliding traction can be applied in many ways, but the principle is always the same. It allows the patient to move about the bed or to move the limb whilst the traction continues to act in the desired line (Fig. 5.4).

Common types of sliding traction

1 Simple traction. This is applied as in Figure 5.4, usually to the skin. It is useful for many conditions, but particularly for those affecting the hip.

2 Longitudinal traction. This is used, for example, for fractures of the femur. It is an alternative to the use of the Thomas' splint as a fixed traction device. The traction is applied through a pin in the upper tibia and the leg is supported on the Thomas' splint with a special knee attachment (Pearson) to allow the knee to be flexed (Fig. 5.5). The splint is usually suspended by cords from an overhead beam. If the tibia is also fractured, this may be immobilized in a below-knee plaster-cast incorporating the tibial pin.

3 Hamilton–Russell traction. This was designed to apply a traction force in line with the shaft of the femur whilst allowing movement of the hip and knee. This is achieved by applying a pull in two directions, giving a resultant force in the desired line in all positions of the limb. It is usually applied with skin extensions and is mainly used for hip conditions and fractures of the upper femur (Fig. 5.6).

4 'Gallows' traction (Bryant). This is a simple method (Fig. 5.7) of applying longitudinal traction to the femur in a child up to the age of 2 years. In older children vascular complications may occur. The traction is arranged to raise the buttocks just clear of the bed.

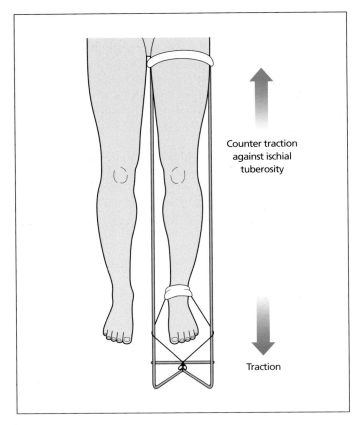

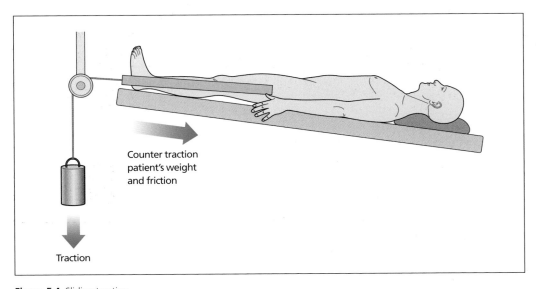

Figure 5.3 Thomas' splint with fixed traction.

Figure 5.4 Sliding traction.

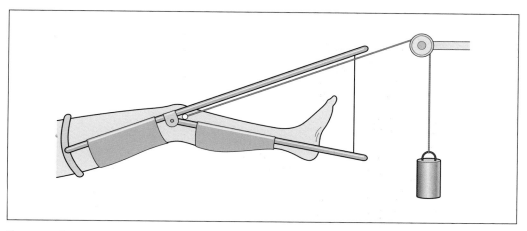

Figure 5.5 Thomas' splint with knee attachment and skeletal traction.

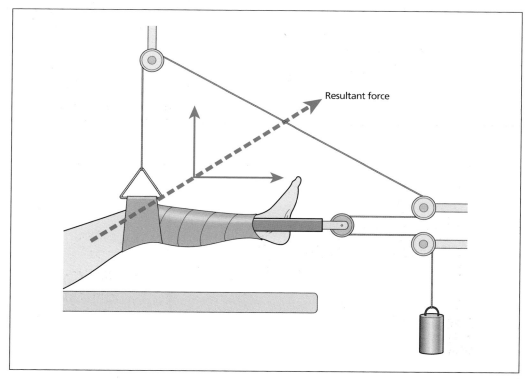

Resultant force

Figure 5.6 Hamilton–Russell traction.

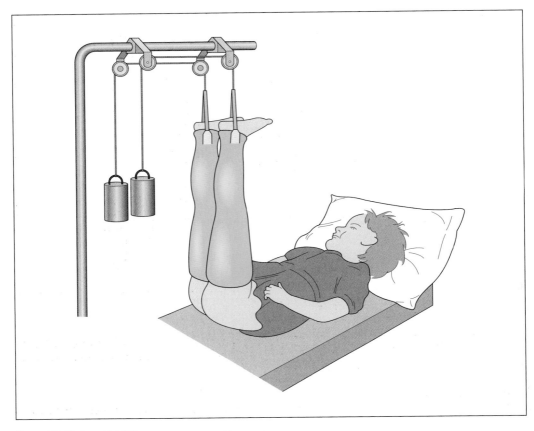

Figure 5.7 'Gallows' traction.

5 Sliding traction using the Böhler–Braun frame. This is a useful method for applying traction to a tibial or femoral fracture. The leg is supported in good alignment on slings stretched across the frame (Fig. 5.8).

Internal fixation

Bony stability promotes soft-tissue healing

Modern fracture management focuses on healing of the soft-tissue damage as well as the fracture itself. Soft tissues heal better with a stable and reduced fracture providing soft-tissue stability also. With this in mind, internal fixation has become more popular as techniques have improved. Fixation is necessary for those fractures where accurate reduction is necessary and when mobilization of the limb or the patient is particularly important. Accurate reduction is essential for fractures involving joint surfaces. Internal fixation can be used, but with more danger due to infection, in open fractures.

Many types of internal fixation device are used: screws, plates, compression plates, intramedullary nails, etc. (Boxes 5.3 and 5.4). The latest techniques utilize advanced engineering principles, and scientifically designed implants, usually arranged to allow some sharing of the load between the bone and the device. Until the 1990s fixation was considered ideal if it was rigid, which required primary bone healing without the formation of callus (see Chapter 4). There is currently interest in internal fixation devices which allow a degree of flexibility

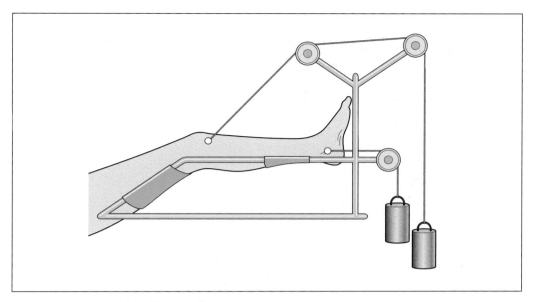

Figure 5.8 Traction using the Böhler–Braun frame.

Box 5.3 Internal fixation—advantages.

- Allows accurate reduction and maintenance of position
- Allows the patient and his/her joints more mobility, thus encouraging rehabilitation and avoiding joint stiffness
- May encourage union, but only if sufficiently strong
- Diminishes time spent in hospital

Box 5.4 Internal fixation—disadvantages.

- May introduce infection
- Is technically exacting and operative complications may occur
- If it is inadequate or infection occurs, union may be long delayed or may not occur
- May not be sufficiently strong to allow the advantages of full mobilization
- Excessively rigid fixation and periosteal stripping may delay union
- Further surgery may be needed to remove the device

---

at the fracture site. The idea is that this may restore some of the natural processes of fracture healing, which can be inhibited by rigid devices. State of the art fixation involves minimal soft-tissue dissection, thus preserving as much blood supply as possible, with devices placed through small incisions and which allow load sharing.

Common techniques of internal fixation

Screw fixation

Simple screw fixation is usually used to attach small bony fragments, e.g. the malleoli. The screw may have a large self-tapping thread which is wider than the shank to give a good grip on cancellous bone (Fig. 5.9), or it may be designed with a standard thread, in which case it is usually necessary to screw into the opposite cortex. This type of screw may be self-tapping, but in most designs (e.g. the AO/ASIF technique) the holes are tapped. A single screw placed at right angles to the fracture line can be used to compress the fracture provided the thread is arranged to bite only into the farther fragment (Fig. 5.10). Such a screw is not in itself sufficient to hold the fracture and a plate or some form of external fixation is required in addition.

Plate fixation

Many sizes and shapes of plate are used to hold fractures. The plate can be designed to apply

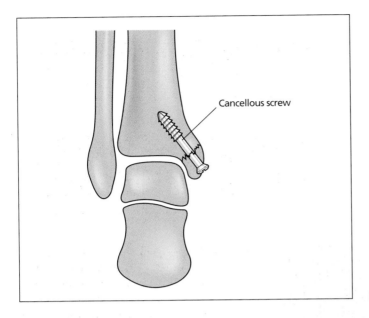

Figure 5.9 Screw fixation.

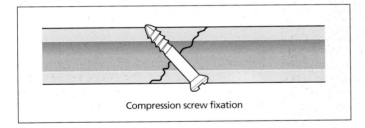

Compression screw fixation

Figure 5.10 Single screw fracture compression.

compression to the fracture in order to give firmer fixation. The shape of the screw heads and the walls of the slot are designed to ensure this in 'dynamic compression plates' (Fig. 5.11).

Intramedullary nail

This technique involves the passage of a rod into the medullary canal of a long bone and across the fracture site, thus stabilizing it in bending. With modern designs these can be introduced distant to the fracture site and through small incisions.

Rotation at the fracture site may happen, especially if the medullary canal is large, and the fragments may slide along the nail, opening a fracture gap or causing the nail to back out. To overcome these problems, the 'locked' nail has been devised. This allows for the insertion through the nail of cross bolts at the upper and lower ends of the shaft (Fig. 5.12). These nails give quite firm fixation but allow small movement at the fracture site which promotes healing by callus. If desired, the screws can be removed from one end of the bone when the fracture becomes reasonably stable, to allow some degree of 'telescoping', which may help to stimulate union, known as dynamizing the fracture. Some nails have the locking bolts passing through slots rather than holes in the nail to allow the fracture to dynamize on weight-bearing.

There is much debate about whether reaming out the medullary canal to allow passage of a larger

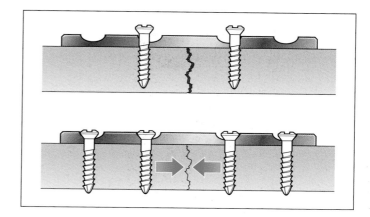

Figure 5.11 Compression plating.

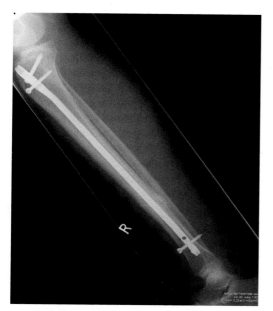

Figure 5.12 Locked intramedullary nail.

nail harms or enhances bone union. Some bones seem more susceptible to non-union following damage to the endosteal (intramedullary) blood supply, such as the tibia, whilst the femur seems more forgiving. This is likely to be related to the degree of soft-tissue coverage.

Long bone fractures in multiply injured patients are best managed by early stabilization and nails are often used for this. This has been shown to reduce mortality.

Infection following intramedullary nailing is usually more difficult to treat than with other methods of internal fixation. If infection occurs, the nail is removed, the medullary canal is then reamed to debride the infection and the bone re-nailed; this is known as exchange nailing. Intramedullary nailing is used mainly in the femur and tibia, less frequently in the humerus.

Wires

These are occasionally used to hold bone fragments in position, e.g. stiff Kirschner wires for Colles fractures or as a figure of 8 tension band wire in olecranon or patella fractures (Fig. 5.13).

Frame fixation

There are situations where external splintage using plaster of Paris or traction may not be adequate or may have other disadvantages, but, on the other hand, internal fixation may be hazardous or technically impossible. In these circumstances, it may be possible to insert pins or fine wires into the bones above and below the fracture and connect these together rigidly by means of a frame assembly (Fig. 5.14). There are many designs of such frames, both for general use and for specific purposes, such as fractures of the pelvis. They have the advantage of giving good fixation whilst allowing access to the fracture site. This may be important if there is a wound requiring attention. They also avoid the dangers of introducing foreign material

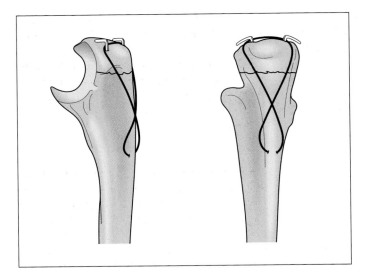

Figure 5.13 Wire fixation of olecranon fracture.

into the fracture site. Frames can be sub-grouped into those with large screws into the bone which have are a bar on one side of the bone—*monolateral fixator*, and those with multiple fine wires through the bone which are then joined to rings around the bone—*circular frames*. Monolateral fixators tend to be expensive and rather clumsy for general use. Furthermore, there is some evidence that rigid fixation of this type, if maintained for too long, may inhibit union, and the frame is often used until the fracture appears stable and is then replaced by a cast. Circular frames allow some movement at the fracture site, whilst still maintaining overall stability, and are very versatile. Circular frames were initially developed in Russia by a surgeon called Ilizarov whose name is often associated with their use (Fig. 5.14). Angular deformities and limb shortening can be managed by the use of external fixators.

Key points

Fracture fixation should be used in the following situations:

1 When adequate reduction cannot be maintained by external splintage (frequently fractures involving joint surfaces)

2 When it is important to allow early movement of a limb or a joint

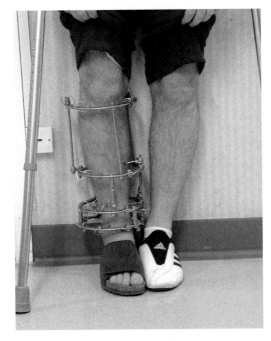

Figure 5.14 Circular frame (Ilizarov).

3 When it is important to avoid a long period of immobilization in bed, e.g. the elderly patient with a femoral neck fracture

4 In cases of multiple trauma, where internal or external fixation of one or more of the fractures

may simplify treatment of other injuries and has been shown to reduce mortality. A fracture associated with a severe vascular injury requiring repair may well come into this category
5 Certain pathological fractures, particularly those resulting from malignancy, where union may be uncertain and the patient's life-expectancy may be short.

With many fractures these criteria do not apply, and closed techniques are perfectly adequate to secure good results.

How long should fixation be maintained?

Fractures vary in the length of time needed for union. Most fractures of the shafts of long bones in adults take at least 12 weeks to unite. Fractures in the cancellous ends of the long bones and in short bones take from 6 to 8 weeks.

In children the times are proportionately reduced with age down to 2–3 weeks for a fracture of the shaft of a long bone in a baby.

If fixation has been used simply to relieve pain rather than to hold an unstable position, it will usually be possible to discard it after 2–3 weeks in an adult and less in a child.

Rehabilitation

This begins immediately after the primary treatment. The limb is moved and used as much as the method of fixation allows. This helps to stimulate union and to prevent joint stiffness. Internal fixation, if secure, has great advantages in this respect. It is also an advantage if the patient can return to his or her normal occupation whilst healing is occurring. When splintage is discontinued, a further period of exercises or physiotherapy is often necessary before full joint function is restored.

Chapter 6

Complications of fractures

Complications are considered by:

1 Time of complication—immediate, intermediate and late

2 Site of complication—general or local

3 Complications specific to the fracture healing.

Time of complication

Immediate complications (i.e. occurring at the time of injury)

General

1 Shock from severe haemorrhage either:
- External
- Internal.

2 Injury to important internal organs—brain, lung, liver, etc.

Local

1 Injury to local nerves or vessels.

2 Skin loss or damage.

Intermediate complications (i.e. occurring during the period of treatment)

General

1 **Deep vein thrombosis and pulmonary embolism.** The former may occur in the immobilized leg

---

Lecture Notes: Orthopaedics and Fractures, 4e.
By T Duckworth and CM Blundell. Published 2010 by Blackwell Publishing.

or elsewhere. It is commoner in patients confined to bed. There is no general agreement as to the best form of prophylaxis. Many patients with hip fractures, for example, receive low molecular weight heparin or aspirin.

2 **Chest infection.**

3 **Renal calculus, acute retention and other urinary tract problems.**

4 **Fat embolism syndrome,** usually occurring 3–10 days after fractures of long bones, and particularly after major trauma. The cause is unknown. It was originally thought to be caused by fat released into the circulation from the fracture site, but it is now thought to be a metabolic phenomenon associated with a period of circulatory insufficiency. It manifests itself as confusion and respiratory difficulty (often detected by a lowered arterial oxygen tension), and a petechial rash which varies in severity. It may lead to acute respiratory distress syndrome (ARDS). It is sometimes fatal, but its severity can be diminished by correct fluid replacement, early immobilization of the fracture and intensive respiratory care.

5 **'Crush syndrome'**—this is usually associated with extensive soft-tissue damage or ischaemia of a large volume of tissues, e.g. following occlusion of the femoral artery. Its cause is complicated; various factors such as fluid loss, release of toxic materials from the site of damage, and possibly diffuse intravascular coagulation, all contribute to an effect on the kidneys, resulting in acute tubular necrosis with renal failure. It may be prevented by removal

of the damaged tissue before severe renal changes have occurred, e.g. by amputation of the limb. If the renal changes become established, dialysis may be necessary in anticipation of recovery of renal function.

Local

1 Compartment syndrome. This is commonest after tibial fractures where swelling in the tightly bound compartments causes venous engorgement in the compartment, further raising pressure and subsequently causing muscle necrosis. This presents as increasing pain some hours after the injury, and paraesthesia and pain on passive movement of the toes. Loss of arterial pulses is a late sign. If suspected, surgical decompression of the compartments is a mandatory emergency (see Chapter 2, p. 18).

2 Gangrene from vascular damage or external pressure.

3 Pressure sores and nerve palsies from splintage or traction.

4 Infection and wound breakdown.

5 Loss of alignment. Failure of internal fixation (Fig. 6.1).

6 Tetanus and gas gangrene.

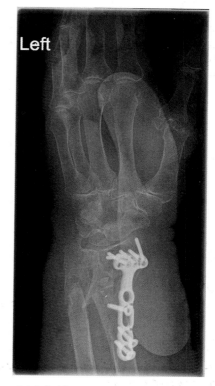

Figure 6.1 Failed fixation of a wrist fracture.

Late complications

General

Post-traumatic psychological disturbances.

Local

1 Delayed and non-union. Malunion, i.e. union in a bad position (see below).

2 Late wound sepsis with skin breakdown.

3 Failure of internal fixation, e.g. breakage or cutting out of plates or nails (Fig. 6.1).

4 Joint stiffness and contracture.

5 Regional pain syndrome (previously variously known as reflex sympathetic dystrophy, Sudek's atrophy or algodystrophy)—a condition in which the limb becomes painful, swollen and discoloured, with obvious circulatory changes and X-rays showing diffuse, patchy porosis of the bones. It is thought to be due to a sympathetic malfunction, but is ill-understood. It appears to be precipitated by trauma, either external or surgical. It is a distressing condition, but usually settles after several weeks or months. During this period it is important that the patient understands the condition and is encouraged to exercise the limb. There is evidence that treatment with calcitonin and sympathetic nerve blocks may shorten the course of the condition in some patients. Neuro-modifying drugs are frequently used, such as gabapentin.

6 Osteoarthritis resulting from joint damage or occasionally from malaligment of the limb.

Complications of fracture healing

The decision as to whether a fracture is united or not is essentially a clinical one: it depends on the disappearance of the original signs of the fracture, i.e. pain, tenderness, abnormal mobility, swelling, etc. Once a fracture is stable, most of these signs diminish. There is usually some residual loss of function after a period of immobilization, so this is not a helpful physical sign in diagnosing union where limbs have been immobilized.

X-rays are helpful in that they may show callus (Fig. 6.2a). This may be visible as early as 3 weeks after a shaft fracture, but when rigid internal fixation is used, callus may be minimal. Even profuse callus may not mean that the fracture is stable, but it is usually an indication that union is proceeding. It can be difficult to assess whether movement is still occurring, but for lower limb fractures significant pain on weight-bearing suggests instability.

Delayed union

Absence of callus with mobility at the fracture site is an indication of delayed union. This means delay beyond the normal time which would normally be expected for the fracture to unite, but still with the possibility of union if immobilization is continued. When the fracture has been rigidly fixed with plates, it may be difficult to judge when union has occurred on clinical and radiological grounds, and the decision to allow unprotected load-bearing may have to be made on the basis of average union times. Occasionally, this leads to load-bearing on a non-united fracture and in these circumstances the fixation device will usually break or cut out of the bone.

Many fractures take longer to unite than the average times suggested (see Chapter 5, p. 43), and protection may still be needed from full load-bearing beyond these times, even though union may apparently have occurred.

Non-union

Non-union, like union, is a clinical and radiological diagnosis. It is commoner in open fractures, infected fractures and characteristic fracture types in which there is poor blood supply, such as the scaphoid bone. Usually the X-ray shows an obvious gap between the bone ends (Fig. 6.2b). True radiological union, characterized by trabeculae crossing the fracture site, is often not evident until long after clinical union has occurred and remodelling may continue for many months after that (Fig. 6.2c). Non-union is commoner with fractures through cortical bone than with fractures of cancellous bone which are often impacted.

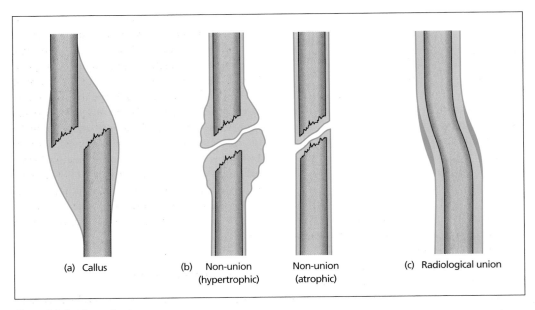

(a) Callus   (b) Non-union (hypertrophic)   Non-union (atrophic)   (c) Radiological union

Figure 6.2 Problems of union.

A decision to treat delayed union is usually made before true non-union occurs. It is usually apparent after 4–5 months that union is not occurring, but in most cases the decision can be made long before this.

Malunion

This expression means that the fracture has united in an unsatisfactory position from either a functional or cosmetic point of view. It should not occur if management of the fracture has been adequate, but circumstances are not always favourable and some patients are left with a degree of deformity or shortening of the limb. In children, considerable compensatory remodelling can be expected and even length defects often correct by the end of growth. In adults, much less correction can be expected, although when the swelling and thickening associated with the fracture have settled, the appearance may be much more satisfactory than might at first have been expected. In some cases, a corrective osteotomy or even bone lengthening with an external fixator may have to be considered. This is a hazardous procedure and in most cases shortness, which is usually only a problem in the lower limb, can be compensated for by modifications to the shoes.

Treatment of delayed or non-union

The management depends on whether the non-union is infected or not. An infected non-union usually fails to heal on antibiotic treatment alone because of the presence of dead bone, either as a separate fragment (sequestrum) or still attached to the living bone.

Non-infected fracture

Non-union is sometimes classified as:
1 **Hypertrophic**, i.e. with much callus at the bone ends, often as a result of excessive fracture site mobility (Fig. 6.2b) or
2 **Atrophic**, i.e. with no obvious callus, often as a result of poor blood supply to the fracture site (Fig. 6.2b).

The hypertrophic type will often unite if the fracture is rigidly immobilized, usually by fixation, e.g. by a plate, nail or external fixator. A compression plate gives particularly firm fixation.

The atrophic non-union also requires firm fixation, but healing tends to proceed more quickly if a bone graft is used to stimulate bone formation. Bone graft (if from the patient it is an autograft) is usually taken from the iliac crest. Bone graft serves a number of functions: induces dormant cells to produce bone (osteo-induction), provides a scaffold over which new bone forms (osteo-conduction) and can provide structural support for bone defects. Harvest of bone graft from the iliac crest is often painful for the patient.

Recently, much interest has been shown in the use of synthetically derived bone morphogenic proteins (BMP), which can be introduced into non-unions to promote union. They have been shown to be as effective as autograft in some situations. Their use is still being evaluated and currently they are very expensive, but it is likely that they will become more extensively used and thus cheaper in the future.

Infected fracture

Union will rarely occur until the infection is overcome. Firm fixation of the fracture and excision of bone which is obviously dead will often eliminate or reduce the infection, enabling a subsequent bone graft to be carried out. If the defect after removal of dead tissue is large, a considerable quantity of bone may be needed to bridge the gap. Immobilization of the fracture needs to be continued until solid union occurs. In severely infected non-unions, an external fixation frame, devised by Ilizarov, is safer than implanting metal plates or nails (see Fig. 5.14). Securing union in such cases can take many months or even years, and in some patients amputation may be a better option.

Factors influencing union

1 **Age.** This is a favourable factor in children, especially young children and babies. In adults, age

affects union very little, even into old age, unless the patient is severely malnourished.

2 Fracture site. Here the important feature is usually the blood supply, especially when one fragment is rendered avascular by the fracture, e.g. scaphoid and femoral neck fractures.

3 Degree of violence. Comminuted fractures with much soft-tissue damage can be expected to unite slowly.

4 Infection. Severe infection, with osteomyelitis, usually delays union.

5 Immobilization—some fractures need more immobilization than others. Fractures of the clavicle, for example, usually unite rapidly with minimal immobilization. In the early stages fol-

lowing the injury, excessively rigid fixation may delay union, but rigid fixation is often used later as a method of treating delayed union.

6 Bone or generalized disease. Local pathology may prejudice union, e.g. malignant disease or infection. Generalized bone disease may or may not matter, e.g. osteoporosis does not necessarily impair healing. Severe malnutrition, vitamin deficiency or steroid excess may interfere with union.

7 Distraction of the bone ends is harmful and is usually avoidable. Interposition of soft tissue may delay or prevent union. If there is evidence that the bone ends are being held apart by soft tissues, it is usually advisable to carry out an open reduction (but not necessarily internal fixation).

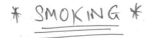
✱ SMOKING ✱

Chapter 7

Major trauma

Major trauma, that is serious, life-threatening injury, is increasing in frequency. This is due in part to greater protection in vehicles, leading to higher survival rates in what would previously have been fatal accidents, and in part to the increase in violent crime. Most patients with multiple injuries have major orthopaedic injuries which in isolation or in combination are life-threatening. The management of major trauma differs from center to center. The key to successful management is to have an effective, early system for resuscitating and assessing the patient, coupled with a service allowing rapid and efficient transfer to a large trauma centre offering wide expertise.

Arrangements for *pre-hospital care* vary in different countries. In the UK this is provided by the ambulance service and advanced training is now provided with the PHLS (Pre-Hospital Life Support).

In the *Accident and Emergency Department* the trend is towards highly trained teams of surgeons, anaesthetists and nursing staff. The Advanced Trauma Life Support (ATLS) system of training was developed in 1976 in the USA by an orthopaedic surgeon who lost members of his family when his light aircraft, which he was piloting, crashed in Nebraska. It is now mandatory in the UK for surgical trainees, but the ideals of the ATLS have spread

worldwide. In this system, the patient is managed by a team, with each member carrying out his/her own tasks and with an experienced team leader providing overall supervision. The leader is responsible for pre-planning the activities of each team member. The process follows the following stages:

1 Primary survey
2 Resuscitation
3 Secondary survey
4 Review, documentation and initial treatment plan.

Primary survey and resuscitation

The primary survey is a sequence of steps from A to E, and the team member is only able to move from one step to the next when the preceding one had been completed. These steps are:

A – **Airway with cervical spine control.** The adequacy of the airway is checked whilst respecting the potential for there being a cervical spine injury by maintaining cervical spine immobilization

B – **Breathing.** The patient needs to be adequately ventilating via the patent airway

C – **Circulation.** There must be a satisfactory volume within the circulation and an adequate cardiac output with control of blood loss

D – **Disability.** A brief assessment of neurological disability

Lecture Notes: Orthopaedics and Fractures, 4e.
By T Duckworth and CM Blundell. Published 2010 by Blackwell Publishing.

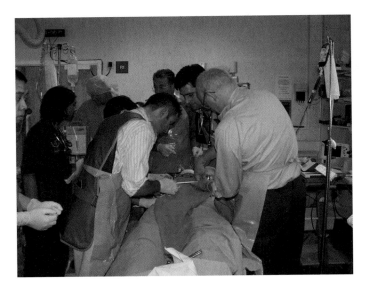

Figure 7.1 Team approach to a major trauma situation.

E – Exposure. The whole patient must be exposed so that any occult injury can be dealt with.

Resuscitation occurs whilst the survey is being carried out, so that at the end of the primary survey the patient should have a stable airway and circulation and be adequately oxygenated. In the multiply injured patient there are often procedures required as the primary survey is being carried out. Each team member has a separate role.

Member 1 is responsible for looking after the 'head end' of the patient and secures the airway, controls and stabilizes the cervical spine, and assesses and assists breathing and oxygenation.

Member 2 is responsible for the circulation and should secure at least two good intravenous lines, assess for the presence of shock, commence fluid resuscitation, take blood for crossmatching, obtain blood gases and ensure external haemorrhage has been controlled.

Member 3 is responsible for carrying out any urgent surgical procedures, such as cricothyroidotomy, chest drainage, intravenous cut-down, etc, which may be needed as judged by the other team members, and for identifying and controlling life-threatening bleeding.

Figure 7.1 shows the team approach to major injury managed in a trauma centre.

Secondary survey

While these procedures are being carried out the team leader is responsible, helped by information from the other team members, for the secondary survey which involves a complete and systematic examination of the patient from head to toe and from front to back, the patient being log-rolled as necessary. At this stage, the level of consciousness is assessed according to the Glasgow coma scale (Table 7.1). X-rays of the cervical spine, chest and pelvis are performed routinely.

Review, documentation and initial treatment plan

The team leader is also responsible for the final review, documentation and initial treatment plan. This involves checking that all resuscitation procedures have been carried out. Sometimes the patient cannot be stabilized and needs to go to theatre immediately for the control of haemorrhage, or alternatively urgent investigation, such as abdominal computed tomography (CT) scanning, are necessary to confirm or rule out life-threatening haemorrhage. A plan is prepared for the further management of the patient and transfer is arranged as necessary.

Table 7.1 Glasgow coma scale.

Verbal response	Orientated	5
	Confused conversation	4
	Inappropriate words	3
	Incomprehensible sounds	2
	Nil	1
Motor function	Obeys	5
	Localizes	4
	Withdraws	3
	Abnormal flexion	3
	Extends	2
	Nil	1
Eye opening	Spontaneous	4
	To speech	3
	To pain	2
	Nil	1

Detailed documentation of the history, physical condition of the patient and all steps taken is carried out before the patient leaves the department.

Many patients require the attention of more than one surgeon for their definitive treatment and it is the duty of the team leader to co-ordinate the activities of the various experts. There are often multiple fractures and joint injuries, and experience has demonstrated that for this type of patient early long bone stabilization gives the best prognosis both for survival and for the injuries themselves.

Trauma care is a constantly changing and advancing area of practice. Those responsible for the care of those who have suffered major injuries must remain abreast of current skills and recommendations, such as those of the ATLS as published by the American College of Surgeons.

Chapter 8

Congenital and developmental conditions

Principles

Many congenital malformations occur for no obvious reasons, but certain factors are known to cause maldevelopment of the fetus if they act at a time when development is at a critical stage.

1 **Genetic disturbances** may be:
  - Inherited or
  - Due to mutations. These may arise spontaneously or as a result of external influences such as radiation.

2 **Drugs**. Thalidomide is the best known example of this, but many others are known, including alcohol.

3 **Infections**. Syphilis is an example of a bacterial and rubella an example of a viral infection which may affect the fetus.

4 **Trauma**. Injury to the baby during labour may produce abnormalities, such as brachial plexus damage or cerebral palsy.

5 **Anoxia**. This may occur during intrauterine life, e.g. as a result of placental separation, or in the immediate postnatal period.

6 **Compression _in utero_**. There has long been debate about compression as a factor in producing malformations of the limbs, such as club foot. A baby with an intrauterine paralytic condition,

such as spina bifida, may fail to make the normal intrauterine movements, so that pressure effects may contribute to the eventual deformities.

Developmental dysplasia of the hip

The term congenital dislocation of the hip (CDH) has been replaced by developmental dysplasia of the hip (DDH) because the latter is more representative and encompasses the spectrum of abnormalities seen in this condition.

Pathology

Capsular laxity is the dominant feature in the unstable hip and the tight fit between the femoral head and acetabulum is lost. The femoral head can be made to slide in and out of the acetabulum.

The primary stimulus for growth and development of the hip joint comes from the femoral head being accurately located in the acetabulum. A possible hypothesis to explain the dysplasia is that the hip will not develop normally unless the head of the femur rotates about a point axis within the acetabulum. If rotation occurs about an eccentric or moveable axis, as in DDH, acetabular development will not proceed normally.

Causes

The cause of the condition is unknown. Girls are affected more than boys (8:1).

Lecture Notes: Orthopaedics and Fractures, 4e.
By T Duckworth and CM Blundell. Published 2010 by Blackwell Publishing.

1 Hereditary factors. The risk is increased to 36% if one parent had DDH. Familial joint laxity may also be a factor in some cases.

2 Environment. The usual incidence is quoted as 1.5 per 1000 live births, but this varies around the world. This may be due to genetic differences or to differences in the way the newborn child is nursed. In those societies where it is usual to nurse the child with the legs bound together in adduction, the incidence of established DDH is much higher than in those societies where the child is carried on the mother's back with the legs widely abducted. It may be that the birth incidence is the same in both groups but that in the second group, the position of carrying the child actually treats the lax hips.

3 Position *in utero*. Breech delivery is more commonly associated with DDH. It is likely that joint laxity is the primary factor and that the vulnerable hip is dislocated by malposition either before or after birth.

Diagnosis

At birth

Clinical examination is crucial. Ortolani and Barlow's manoeuvres are carried out.

The baby is examined when warm and comfortable, preferably after a feed. The baby lies supine and the examiner holds the legs with the hips and knees flexed and the fingertips behind the hip joint and thumb in front, so that the femoral head is between the fingers and thumb (Fig. 8.1). The legs are gradually abducted from the together position and the range of abduction noted. The normal hip in a neonate will abduct until the outside of the thigh lies flat on the couch (Fig. 8.2).

If Ortolani's sign is positive there may be slight limitation of abduction and as the hip is abducted the head slips over the edge of the acetabulum into the joint with a clunk. In other words, the head is out of joint in adduction but slips in easily in abduction.

With the child supine as before, the examiner adducts the leg with the hip and knee flexed. If Barlow's sign is positive, the femoral head is palpated as it exits the acetabulum partially or completely. Over the last few years there has been

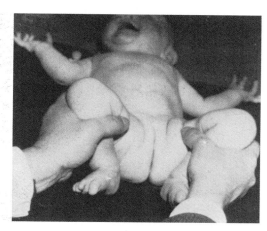

Figure 8.1 Barlow's test for hip instability.

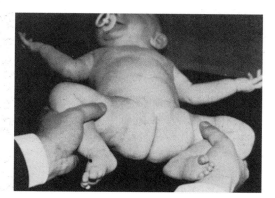

Figure 8.2 Barlow's test showing full abduction.

increasing concern about the failure of clinical examination (screening) to reduce the incidence of late diagnosed DDH. Clinical examination requires experience to obtain consistent results. It is the view of many that in some cases which were diagnosed late, the hip was either normal when examined at birth or the standard tests are not sensitive enough. This had led to a search for more objective tests and particularly to the use of ultrasonography. Ultrasonography demonstrates soft tissues, including articular cartilage. It also allows dynamic screening to ascertain the movement of the femoral head in relationship to the acetabulum. Radiographs are of no use in the neonatal period.

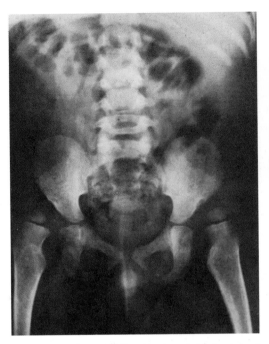

Figure 8.3 Radiograph of late developmental dysplasia of the hip.

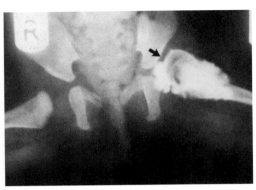

Figure 8.4 Arthrogram of a case of late developmental dysplasia of the hip; arrow points to the limbus.

Later in life

The leg may be short and abduction of the hip limited. The femoral head may be felt to move in and out of the joint in abduction, or may fail to reduce and be palpable in the buttock. Most late cases are spotted when the child walks. The child usually walks with a characteristic waddle (Trendelenburg gait) due to inefficiency of the abductor muscles.

X-rays usually make the diagnosis obvious (Fig. 8.3). An arthrogram, in which radio-opaque dye is injected into the joint, will show the exact position and shape of the head and may show the inverted capsule (limbus) (Fig. 8.4). It is likely, however, that MRI scanning will replace arthrography as the investigation of choice.

Treatment

The principles of treatment are to reduce the hip and maintain reduction, thus providing an optimum environment for development of the femoral head and acetabulum. This is the same irrespective of the age of the child. The older the child when the diagnosis is made, the more difficult it is to achieve the treatment goals.

Newborns and infants less than 6 months of age

Treatment must begin as soon as the diagnosis is made (after birth). There is no place for the use of double or triple nappies.

Splinting the limb in abduction usually allows reduction and stabilization of the hip. The Pavlik harness is the most commonly used device in the newborn period but others, such as the Von Rosen splint and Frejka pillow, are available.

The Pavlik harness may be used until the age of 6 months (Fig 8.5). Application of the harness must be shown to the family members and a child in a harness must be reviewed at regular intervals. Clinical examination is necessary to check the progress of treatment and ultrasonography may also be used.

Children 6 months to 2 years of age

In children older than 6 months at diagnosis and those who have failed a trial of Pavlik harness, closed reduction is indicated. This procedure is carried out under general anaesthesia and in the operating room. The proximal femoral head is gently manipulated into the acetabulum by applying traction with flexion and abduction. An arthrogram is undertaken to confirm reduction. An open or percutaneous adductor tenotomy is necessary in most cases. If reduction is achieved, it is maintained by applying a moulded plaster-cast hip spica (Fig. 8.6) or abduction cylinders (Fig. 8.7). The time in cast varies but is usually about 3 months, with a cast change at 6 weeks in the operating room. If closed treatment fails to achieve reduction, open reduction is indicated.

There are usually several obstacles to reduction (Fig. 8.8):

1 The glenoid labrum and superior capsule may be folded inwards to form a concentric flap—this is called the limbus

2 The psoas tendon may constrict the inferior capsule like an hour glass

3 The inferior capsule may be infolded and adherent to the floor of the true acetabulum

4 The ligamentum teres may be hypertrophied.

The operation consists of opening the capsule, dividing the psoas and inferior capsule and, if possible, reducing the head under the limbs into the true acetabulum. The redundant capsule may need to be tightened. A moulded plaster-cast hip spica is applied.

Children older than 2 years of age

Open reduction is usually necessary if the diagnosis of DDH is made in children aged 2 years or older. A femoral shortening osteotomy may be required to achieve reduction of the hip joint. Depending on the stability of the reduction, an acetabular osteotomy may be necessary at the time of the open reduction or at a later date.

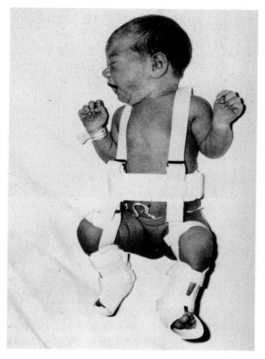

Figure 8.5 Pavlik harness.

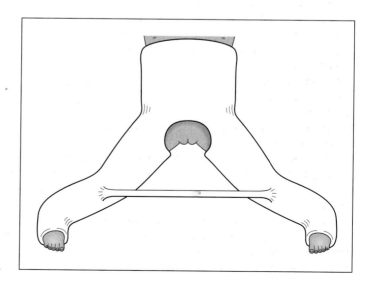

Figure 8.6 Internal rotation hip spica.

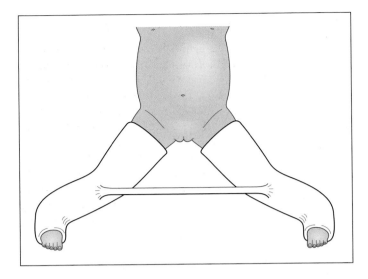

Figure 8.7 Abduction cylinders.

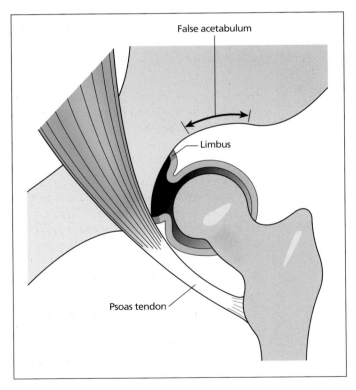

Figure 8.8 Obstacles to reduction of late developmental dysplasia of the hip.

Avascular necrosis of the femoral head is a recognized complication of treatment, especially if forcible manipulation is used.

Knee deformities

Recurrent dislocation of the patella

This is a relatively common condition, typically affecting adolescent girls. The patella dislocates laterally, often as a result of an accident. Subsequently, dislocation occurs relatively easily. The complaint is often that the knee locks in flexion. When this happens it may not be noticed that the patella is dislocated or it may have been 'knocked back' easily, allowing the knee to extend. The knee is usually normal between attacks. The condition may be associated with generalized joint laxity or a malalignment of the tibial tubercle. Rarely, and usually in younger children, it is associated with contracture of the quadriceps muscles, particularly the vastus lateralis. In some cases this appears to have been caused by repeated intramuscular injections for an illness in infancy. In these cases the patella dislocates each time the knee is flexed.

In the ordinary idiopathic variety, a useful clinical sign, indeed often the only sign, is a tendency for the patient to be apprehensive when the patella is pushed laterally. 'Skyline' X-rays may show an abnormal tilt of the patella or a defect of the lateral femoral condyle. The patella may be small and placed rather higher than usual.

Treatment

The recurrent case is often treated by transplantation of the patellar tendon more medially. If the child is near to maturity, this is usually done by transplanting a block of bone bearing the insertion of the tendon to a more medial and distal position on the tibia. The operation is usually successful in preventing dislocation, but there is increasing evidence that it may be followed by osteoarthritis in later life. The younger child may require a release of the tight vastus lateralis combined with 'reefing' of the medial capsule.

Genu valgum—knock knee

Many children have valgus knees when they first walk. These usually start to correct spontaneously by the age of 6, provided there is no underlying cause such as rickets, epiphyseal dysplasia, etc.

Rarely, the condition starts late or persists, is ugly and may predispose to osteoarthritis in adult life. If the condition is still troublesome at the age of 11 or 12, it may be corrected easily by inserting staples across the inner side of the femoral or both the femoral and tibial epiphyses. These slow down growth on that side and the knee gradually straightens. Slight over-correction is allowed, and the staples are then removed.

Tibia vara (Blount's disease)

This is a rare condition in which there is a developmental defect of the medial part of the upper tibial epiphysis, resulting in a progressive bow-leg deformity. This may be unilateral or bilateral. The deformity may become very severe. It is more common in black than in white children.

Treatment
Osteotomy of the upper end of the tibia is carried out early to correct deformity. This may need to be repeated during growth.

Pseudarthrosis of the tibia

This is a condition present at birth or developing in early childhood in which bowing of the tibia occurs, often associated with a cystic defect in the lower third and eventually resulting in a fracture which persistently fails to unite. The cause is unknown, but there is an association with neurofibromatosis and possibly with fibrous dysplasia.

Treatment
If the bowing is recognized before the fracture occurs, it may be possible to protect the bone with a plaster-cast or to carry out a bypass bone graft. The established case is usually very resistant to surgery, although firm internal fixation and bone grafting may secure union. The leg may become grossly shortened and require amputation in late childhood.

Congenital dislocation of the knee

This is a very rare condition. The child is born with the knee hyper-extended and with the tibia dislocated anteriorly. Operative reduction may be necessary if stretching and serial plaster-cast immobilization fails.

Discoid meniscus

In this condition the lateral meniscus of the knee fails to develop normally, remaining as a complete disc. Occasionally the medial meniscus is involved. The patient complains of knee joint pain, snapping and swelling. Magnetic resonance imaging (MRI) is useful in confirming the diagnosis and determining if there is an associated meniscal tear, as this type of meniscus is more prone to injury than the normal one. Surgery may be required if the condition is symptomatic and involves a partial meniscectomy, with or without meniscal repair if there is a tear amenable to repair.

Foot deformities

An appreciation of terminology is important to enable a deformity to be described and hence to make a diagnosis.

Equinus—means that the hindfoot is plantar flexed at the ankle.

Calcaneus—the hindfoot is dorsiflexed at the ankle.

Varus—the hindfoot is adducted or inverted when looked at from behind.

Valgus—the hindfoot is abducted or everted when looked at from behind.

Cavus—the longitudinal arch is higher than usual.

Planus—the arch is flattened (and the foot is usually valgus).

In general the forefoot tends to follow the alignment of the hindfoot. When the latter is varus, the sole tends to face medially, i.e. supination, and when the hindfoot is valgus the sole tends to face more laterally than normal, producing a flat foot pronation. The situation may be complicated by the fact that the forefoot may point in a different direction from the hindfoot, e.g. hindfoot neutral or calcaneus, forefoot plantar-flexed. Similarly, the forefoot may be adducted or abducted relative to the hindfoot. In these circumstances it is better to use the full descriptive terms for each part of the foot.

Calcaneo valgus

The baby is born with a foot that is markedly dorsiflexed at the ankle joint and everted at the subtalar joint. The dorsum of the foot is often in contact with the anterior shin. The deformity is thought to be caused by intrauterine malposition/moulding. Passive stretching exercises can be undertaken by the parents and surgery is not required as the prognosis for spontaneous correction is excellent.

Congenital vertical talus or convex pes valgus

Congenital vertical talus is a dorsolateral dislocation of the navicular on the talus (Fig. 8.9). This is a rare deformity. The hindfoot is in a fixed equinovalgus position and the midfoot is dorsiflexed and abducted on the hindfoot, giving the appearance of a Persian slipper.

Treatment

The initial treatment involves manipulation and serial casting, but the corrective forces applied must be opposite to those for talipes equinovarus correction. If this fails to correct the deformity, surgery is required.

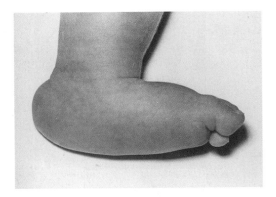

Figure 8.9 Vertical talus deformity.

Metatarsus adductus

Sometimes called metatarsus varus, this condition is characterized by medial deviation of the forefoot on the hindfoot, resulting in the forefoot pointing inwards. The cause is unknown but it may occur as a result of inadequate correction of talipes equinovarus.

Treatment

If severe at birth or when first diagnosed, non-operative measures, including stretching exercises, splints/braces and serial casting, are advised. The severe uncorrected case may require midfoot surgery, but this is rarely indicated.

Congenital talipes equinovarus (club foot)

Congenital talipes equinovarus is characterized by a complex malalignment of the bones and joints of the foot and ankle (Fig. 8.10). The deformities are equinus and inversion of the hindfoot, cavus (plantar flexion of the forefoot on the hindfoot) and adduction of the forefoot on the midfoot so that the sole of the foot points medially or even upwards. The cause is unknown but various theories have been proposed and these include primary muscle, vascular or neurological abnormalities and/or *in utero* moulding. Club feet may be idiopathic, postural, neurogenic or syndromic. It is important to examine the child fully to exclude other associated anomalies. The foot and calf are smaller than the contralateral side in unilateral cases but the condition may be bilateral.

Treatment

Treatment should begin as soon as the diagnosis is made and the goal is to achieve a plantigrade, supple, painless foot. The technique of manipulation and serial casting popularized by Ponsetti *et al* is the gold standard.

Late recurrence may occur up to the age of 4 or even later, and it may then become necessary to correct the residual deformity by bone operations, such as that designed by Evans, in which the calcaneo-cuboid joint is excised to produce a lateral fusion (Fig. 8.11). This partly corrects

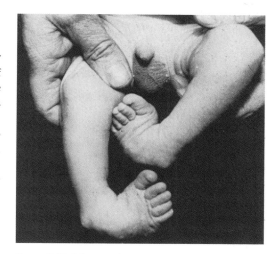

Figure 8.10 Talipes equinovarus.

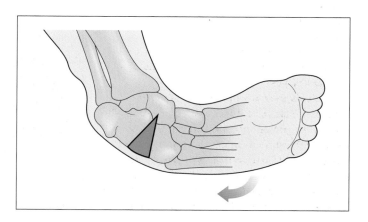

Figure 8.11 Dilwyn Evans operation for relapsed club foot.

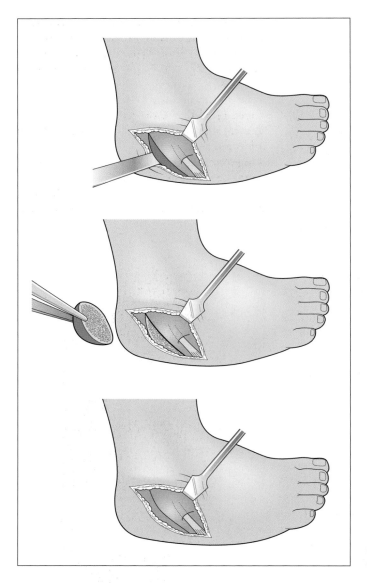

Figure 8.12 Dwyer operation for relapsed club foot.

the deformity and relies on further growth on the inner side to complete the correction. The operation devised by Dwyer concentrates on taking a wedge from the outer side of the os calcis to correct the inversion of the heel. He believes that growth corrects the remaining deformity (Fig. 8.12).

Syndactyly (fusion of digits)

These abnormalities are relatively common. They occur because of a failure of separation of the digits *in utero*. Surgical separation of the affected fingers is usually carried out around the age of 12 months. Syndactyly of the toes does not cause functional limitations and surgery to separate affected toes is not advised.

Upper limb deformities

Madelung's deformity

In this condition the volar ulnar aspect of the distal radial physis fails to develop normally so that the radius becomes bowed with an oblique distal end. In addition, the distal end of the ulna appears prominent.

Madelung's deformity usually occurs in girls and is often bilateral. It may be associated with Turner's syndrome, achondroplasia and Ollier's disease.

Patients presenting with a marked deformity and symptoms require surgery and this involves corrective osteotomies.

Cerebral palsy

This is a disorder of movement and posture resulting from injury to the immature brain. The aetiology includes intrauterine developmental defects, birth trauma, asphyxia and diseases or injuries in early life.

The condition is essentially a motor disorder with a mixture of muscle weakness and spasticity. Initially, a dynamic deformity may be present but persistent spasticity leads to short muscles, contractures, bony deformity, joint subluxation and dislocation. The child may also have additional disabilities, such as mental retardation, sensory abnormalities, speech defects and blindness.

Cerebral palsy is divided into various types based on:
1 **Physiology** (type of movement disorder)
2 **Topography** (geographical distribution).

Physiological classification
1 **Spasticity**—this is an upper motor neurone type defect and is characterized by increased muscle tone and reflexes. This is the common form of cerebral palsy.

2 **Ataxia**—this is characterized by an inability to co-ordinate muscles for voluntary movement.
3 **Athetosis**—in this type, the limbs move at random, with jerking and inco-ordinated movements.

Topographic classification
This classification is based on the degree of limb involvement.
1 **Hemiplegia**—the upper and lower limbs on the same side are involved (Fig. 8.13).
2 **Diplegia**—involvement of both lower limbs.
3 **Quadriplegia**—all four limbs are involved (Fig. 8.14).

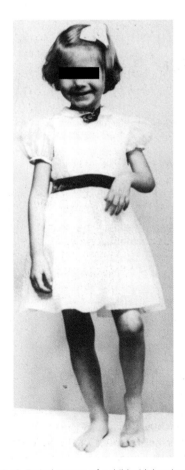

Figure 8.13 Typical posture of a child with hemiparesis.

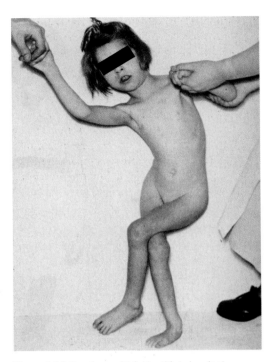

Figure 8.14 Spastic quadriplegia with 'scissoring'.

Management

The first step in the management of a child with cerebral palsy is a thorough history and clinical examination. The child's balance, sitting and gait must also be assessed. Gait analysis is helpful in assessing movement disorder in those children who can walk. The child is usually managed by a team consisting of paediatrians, orthopaedic surgeons, physiotherapists and other specialists as necessary. Treatment must be goal-oriented and may be surgical or non-surgical. Available treatments include physiotherapy, use of orthoses (splints), intramuscular botulinum toxin injection, oral or intradermal baclofen and surgery.

Physiotherapy

Physiotherapy is often the first and commonest modality used.

The aims of physiotherapy are to:

1 Assist assessment
2 Prevent or attempt to correct musculoskeletal deformity
3 Train the child in posture and movement
4 Provide suitable sensory stimulation.

Orthoses

These may help improve gait in those who are ambulatory. They may also be used post-operatively while muscle weakness is being addressed through physiotherapy. Botulinum toxin has been shown to be helpful in weakening muscles that produce dynamic deformities. Unfortunately, its action is temporary and repeated injections may be required.

Surgery

This involves soft tissues and or bony surgery. It is advisable to combine bony and soft-tissue surgery to various parts of the limb in one surgical event rather than to undertake surgery every year as used to be the practice and called 'birthday surgery'.

The aims of surgery are:

1 To correct any established deformity:
  • Soft-tissue surgery involves dividing tendon, capsules, skin, etc. Common procedures are elongation of the gastrocnemius, hamstrings and adductors of the hip
  • Bony correction is needed when deformities are severe, usually with simple osteotomies, e.g. through the lower femur to correct a flexion deformity of the knee.
2 To restore muscle balance and diminish spasticity:
  • Tendon lengthening achieves this to some extent
  • Occasionally, tendons may be transferred, usually in the upper limb.

Physiotherapy is essential after surgery as even minor procedures may interfere severely with function, especially in the older child.

Considerable social and psychological support for the child and family may be necessary.

Spinal malformations

Congenital malformations of the spine are commonest in the lower thoracic, lumbar and sacral regions. Minor malformations of the lumbosacral junction are very common and usually of little significance. Of the more serious deformities, the commonest and most important is spina bifida.

Spinal dysraphism

This is a condition in which the neural arches fail to form or close posteriorly. It is often associated with abnormal development of the spinal cord and meninges. Various degrees of the condition occur.

1 **Spina bifida occulta** is common and usually of no importance (Fig. 8.15a).

2 **Meningocele** is not necessarily associated with cord abnormality but the sac is continuous with the skin and may need excision and closure of the defect (Fig. 8.15b).

3 **Spina bifida with myelomeningocele** is one of the commonest congenital malformations (Fig. 8.15c). It has important clinical consequences:

- The vertebrae themselves, as well as being defective posteriorly, are often malformed, causing serious spinal deformity, such as scoliosis and kyphosis, the latter usually being localized to the thoracolumbar region

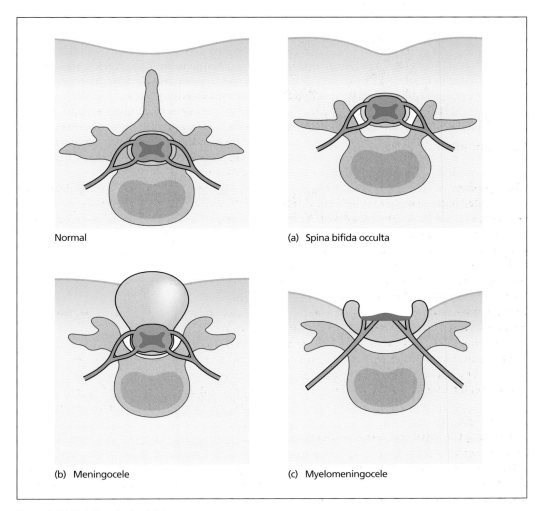

Normal

(a) Spina bifida occulta

(b) Meningocele

(c) Myelomeningocele

Figure 8.15 Varieties of spina bifida.

- The cord is opened out on the surface and is functionally abnormal, resulting in lower limb and possibly trunk paralysis with paralysis of the bladder and anal sphincter
- There is frequently an associated malformation of the brain stem, resulting in hydrocephalus and often mental defect (Arnold–Chiari malformation).

Management

The condition has received much attention since it became apparent that babies with myelomeningocele could be kept alive by closing the spinal defect surgically and that the hydrocephalus could also be controlled. It has become usual for affected babies to be managed in special centres by a paediatric team.

1 A detailed assessment at birth by orthopaedic and neurological surgeons, paediatricians, social workers, etc is essential if an accurate prognosis is to be made. This includes:

- Accurate assessment of deformities, neurological state of the limbs, both motor and sensory
- Assessment of the hydrocephalus
- Assessment of the genitourinary tract.

2 A decision is them made as to whether the spinal defect should be closed surgically. If this is not done, death is usual. Some babies survive for many years, but, if necessary, the defect can then be closed at a later stage. Those babies who have good innervation of the legs are regarded as suitable for urgent closure, i.e. within the first 24 hours, because of the risk of neurological deterioration if closure is delayed.

3 If the hydrocephalus is progressing, a valve may be used to shunt cerebrospinal fluid from the ventricles back to the circulation, usually into a neck vein.

4 Orthopaedic problems. Several consequences stem from paralysis of the legs:

- Deformities may develop due to muscle imbalance. These may affect any of the joints, but particularly the hips and feet
- Activities may be restricted by the motor loss. The joints may lack stability because of muscle weakness

- The limbs may be liable to pressure sores and fractures from lack of normal sensation.

Orthopaedic treatment aims

1 To avoid or correct deformity by splintage or appropriate corrective surgery.
2 To try to secure muscle balance by partial denervation or tendon transfer.
3 To improve mobility by the use of appliances.

Neurosurgical treatment is required for the hydrocephalus and treatment is necessary for the urinary tract and bowel problems. This may involve the control of recurrent infection, diversion of the ureters, sphincter surgery, etc.

The majority of children with spina bifida have severe and multiple disabilities and follow-up is likely to continue indefinitely. The tendency at the moment is to concentrate treatment on those most likely to benefit from it. The problem has diminished recently because of the falling birth rate, the reduction in the prevalence of the condition and improved techniques for prenatal diagnosis, offering the possibility of termination.

Congenital scoliosis

A scoliosis is a lateral curvature of the spine. It is almost always associated with a rotation of the spine. It is uncommon in the neonate. In babies most minor curves improve with growth. The more severe curves and those with structural abnormalities, such as hemi-vertebrae, usually progress and become very severe in later childhood. An attempt is usually made to hold the curve by an external support, such as a Milwaukee brace (Fig. 8.16), but this is of limited value.

Congenital malformations of the cervical spine

These occur infrequently. They include the Klippel–Feil syndrome in which the cervical vertebrae are deformed and often fused so that the neck is shortened and webbed. This is often associated with elevation of one or both scapulae—Sprengel's shoulder.

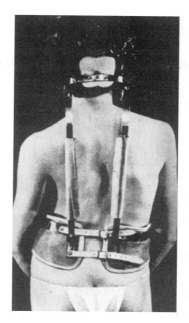 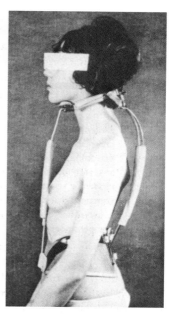

Figure 8.16 Milwaukee brace.

Congenital torticollis

This is a condition in which the child develops a fixed, fusiform swelling in one sternomastoid muscle, usually during the first 2 weeks after birth. The sternomastoid 'tumour' subsides, but the subsequent fibrosis causes a tilt and rotation of the neck to the opposite side. When the condition is well established, the face is usually asymmetrical with the eyes on a different level.

Treatment

Passive stretching in the early stages often prevents deformity. Late uncorrected cases may require surgical release of the sternomastoid. The operation may correct the torticollis, but the asymmetry of the face remains.

Chapter 9

Generalized orthopaedic conditions

Skeletal dysplasias

This is a group of generalized conditions affecting bone and cartilage, which are mostly inherited. Although each is rare, because there are many dysplasias, collectively they are reasonably common. Classification is difficult in such a heterogenous group of disorders. Only the most common are described here, classified according to the principle tissue type involved.

Bone dysplasias

Osteogenesis imperfecta (brittle bone disease)

A connective tissue disease in which the bones are of decreased density, rendering them delicate and prone to fracture. The condition is caused by an abnormality of Type 1 collagen which in the eye allows the blue colour of the retina to show through. Vision is not affected. No treatment is known, but severe cases require protection from everyday injuries. It is possible to protect the long bones from fractures with expanding intramedullary rods which increase in length as the child grows. The tendency to fracture often becomes less in adult life. There are four types:

Lecture Notes: Orthopaedics and Fractures, 4e.
By T Duckworth and CM Blundell. Published 2010 by Blackwell Publishing.

Type 1 Autosomal dominant inheritance. Blue sclerae. This is the commonest group. The teeth are normal in group A, whilst group B have weak teeth.

Type 2 Autosomal recessive inheritance. Dark blue sclerae. There is a high perinatal mortality, often the child is stillborn.

Type 3 Sporadic cases. White sclerae. Progressive deformity with fractures often present at birth.

Type 4 Autosomal dominant inheritance. White sclerae. Osteoporosis and fractures occur. Grouped into A and B as for Type 1.

The severity varies, but patients often have multiple fractures over many years. The fractures heal well but may cause multiple deformities and dwarfism.

Fibrous dysplasia

This is a condition in which single or multiple cystic lesions occur in the bones. The proximal ends of long bones are usually affected and the condition is recognized in early adult life, often by the bone fracturing or occasionally because of swelling or deformity. The defects may be localized or may extend to involve the whole bone; if solitary they are known as monostotic. When the lesions are multiple (polyostotic) they may be associated with endocrine disturbance and pigmented skin patches and are then known as the McCune–Albright syndrome. The lesions are usually radiolucent with scalloped edges and occa-

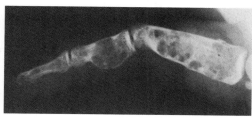

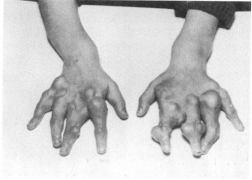

Figure 9.2 Multiple enchondromatosis.

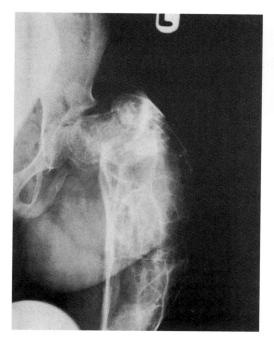

Figure 9.1 Fibrous dysplasia.

sionally expand the bone (Fig. 9.1), but always leave a layer of cortex. Microscopically, they consist of loose cellular tissue with spicules of bone.

Neurofibromatosis (Von Recklinghausen's disease)

This condition is a congenital hamartomatous dysplasia with all cell types affected. In this condition pigmented skin lesions and multiple fibromata in skin and on peripheral nerves are often associated with multiple areas of fibrous dysplasia. In some cases central neuromata and brain tumours, such as astrocytomas, occur. Scoliosis occurs in 30% of cases and, occasionally, localized gigantism of part or the whole of a limb.

Cartilaginous dysplasias

Multiple epiphyseal dysplasia

This is one of the more common dysplasias and is autosomal dominant in some families. The child is usually of short stature, with symmetrically short limbs, and may have difficulty in walking. There may be impaired upper limb function. Affected joints are stiff and occasionally painful, but the number of affected joints varies. The epiphyses ossify late and incompletely, resulting in deformity with apparently wide joint spaces. For example, the femoral head may ossify at 1–2 years, resulting in coxa vara. The vertebrae are usually spared.

Multiple enchondromatosis (Ollier's disease)

This is a non-hereditary disorder of the growth plate, resulting in areas of unossified hyaline cartilage arising around the growth plate area. The condition affects the long bones only and often only one bone. The limb is often shortened with the hands particularly affected. The lesions are found in the metaphyses and tend to increase in size and expand the bone, producing multiple swellings. In adult life, function may be grossly impaired (Fig. 9.2). Treatment usually consists of excising those lesions which are causing trouble, and correcting deformities by osteotomy, so that multiple surgery may be necessary. Malignant change in a lesion, to form a chondrosarcoma, is very rare.

Hereditary multiple exostoses

Also known as diaphyseal aclasia, this is strongly hereditary condition in which the bones develop exostoses of cancellous bone, capped with cartilage and arising from the region of the epiphysis. The exostosis typically points away from the end of the bone due to the direction of long bone growth (Fig. 9.3). Multiple swellings can be palpated and these increase in size with the child. The long bones, iliac crests and scapulae are most usually affected. The swellings may be excised as necessary. The risk of malignancy occurring in adult life is rare and is proportional to the number of lesions.

Achondroplasia

A hereditary condition in 20% of cases (autosomal dominant) and in 80% it occurs sporadically. This is the commonest of the disorders caused by abnormal maturation of growth plate chondroblasts. It is present at birth and most noticeably affects the long bones, resulting in stereotypical dwarfism, so that the individual has a normal trunk but short limbs—The forehead is large and the nose flattened. The hands are short and broad with a short middle finger. Spinal canal stenosis and spinal deformity often lead to abnormal lower limb neurology. X-rays show the bones to be short and dense with flared ends. The acetabulum is broad and flat, and the ilium is quadrilateral. The vertebrae have concave posterior borders and thick, short pedicles. Mental function is normal.

Mucopolysaccharidoses

A group of rare congenital disorders of growth associated with dwarfism, and in some cases mental deficiency. They are caused by a defect of mucopolysaccharide metabolism affecting cartilage matrix formation and resulting in deposition of abnormal mucopolysaccharides in the bones and their excretion in the urine (kerato-sulphate).

Coagulation defects

Haemophilia and related disorders

Haemophilia is a sex-linked recessive disease affecting males only (except on the rare occasions when a marriage between a male patient and a carrier female may produce a female child with the disease). In one-third of cases the disease appears to result from a spontaneous mutation. Haemophilia is the most important defect of the blood clotting mechanism causing orthopaedic problems. In haemophilia A, Factor VIII and in haemophilia B (Christmas disease), Factor IX are deficient in the plasma. The level of Factor VIII may vary from time to time and is given as a percentage of normal. A level below 1% poses a significant risk of spontaneous joint haemorrhages.

Clinical features
The disease may be suspected if there is a history of prolonged or severe bleeding from minor

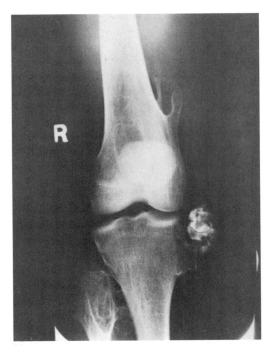

Figure 9.3 Hereditary multiple exostoses.

injuries, with a tendency to develop extreme bruising or swelling. Small wounds such as pin-pricks may not bleed abnormally, but extraction of a tooth may be followed by a dangerous haemorrhage.

Haemorrhages tend to track along fascial planes and fill tissue compartments, and may result in nerve compression or vascular occlusion. Bleeding within the iliacus sheath is a common example of this phenomenon, and is often accompanied by paralysis of the femoral nerve. Median and ulnar palsies are also relatively common, usually associated with bleeds into the forearm muscular compartments.

The main orthopaedic problems are those relating to the development of acute haemarthroses and large intramuscular collections. These occur spontaneously in severe haemophiliacs and are a frequent reason for hospital admission. The knee, elbow and ankle are the commonest joints involved. There may be a definite injury, but in many cases the bleeding appears to be truly spontaneous and may occur during sleep. Haemarthroses tend to be more common in young patients, particularly adolescents.

Recurrent bleeding in the same joint is common and leads to gradual destruction of the articular cartilage, with internal fibrosis and a tendency to develop contractures—haemoarthropathy.

The haemarthroses are usually extremely painful and accompanied by severe muscle spasm. The joint is distended, except in those patients where repeated bleeds have produced so much fibrosis that distension is impossible. There is usually a local increase in temperature, and tenderness over the synovium. In chronic cases the range of movement may be diminished, with almost total destruction of the joint.

Large soft-tissue collections of blood may fail to reabsorb (so called pseudo-tumours) and may, indeed, increase in size, forming cysts which may compress surrounding structures and even penetrate bone.

Diagnosis

The patient is often aware of his condition and may have similarly affected relatives. Approxi-mately one-third of patients however, present for the first time with no family history. These patients require a full and detailed haematological investigation of the clotting factors to assess the precise nature of the defect and its severity.

Treatment and prophylaxis

The mainstay of treatment is replacement of the defective factor. This usually relieves the pain and bleeding dramatically. Factor replacement is also needed in planned orthopaedic procedures which hitherto would have been prohibited by the risks of bleeding. Joint replacement in haemophiliacs is becoming more commonplace.

The factor can be supplied in several forms.

1 Fresh frozen plasma. This can be given as an outpatient procedure, but is most effective within 4 hours of the onset of bleeding.

2 Cryoprecipitate. This material is a cold precipitate of fibrinogen containing considerable Factor VIII activity (but not Factor IX). It can be reconstituted to give a potent preparation.

3 Freeze-dried human AHG (Factor VIII) concentrate. This can be stored for long periods.

4 Animal antihaemophilic globulin.

5 Recombinant tissue factors, artificially created by genetic engineering.

The use of some of these products has been complicated by the transmission of human immunodeficiency virus (HIV) infection to the patients, and since 1986 all blood products are now appropriately treated by heat and screened. Concerns regarding transmission of new variant Creutzfelt Jacob disease (nvCJD) has resulted in the increased usage of recombinant tissue factors; in the UK all Factor VIII given is now recombinant. Since 1998 all children in the UK have been treated with recombinant factors.

A restoration of 15–20% factor level is adequate for most minor to moderate bleeds. Levels of 30% or more may be needed for severe bleeds or bleeds in dangerous situations. At this level of cover, almost any surgical procedure can be carried out.

Acute self-administration of factor therapy reduces the risk of severe bleeding after injury in those with severe disease.

Other aspects of treatment

It is usual to splint the limb which has developed the haemorrhage to prevent further bleeding. Large haemarthroses may be aspirated, with the patient covered by Factor VIII therapy. This appears to reduce the risk of permanent damage to the articular cartilage by the blood in the joint. Cover is needed until bleeding has obviously stopped. After this, the blood usually re-absorbs and the joint becomes comfortable to move. At this point, mobilization can be started, but it is normally necessary to give a further period of cover, particularly if physiotherapy or manipulation is necessary to regain movements. The chronically damaged knee is very prone to repeated bleeds and a caliper or splint may be tried in the hope of diminishing the need for hospitalization and preventing unnecessary damage to the joint.

Nerve palsies are usually treated conservatively, although a severe bleed into a closed fascial space may need surgical decompression.

It should be remembered that, after severe bleeding, transfusion of blood may be necessary for replacement of blood volume, independently of factor replacement. Some patients eventually develop inhibitors in the plasma, and no longer respond to Factor VIII concentrate. At this point, risks from fatal bleeding are much intensified, and many patients die eventually from renal complications.

Paget's disease

Paget's disease is one of the commonest bone diseases, affecting in Great Britain as many as 4% of the population. The disease was originally described by Sir James Paget in 1879 and named by him 'osteitis deformans'.

Distribution

Great Britain and western Europe have the highest world incidence. It is also common in the eastern states of the USA and eastern Australia, where it is almost confined to migrants of British descent. It is almost unknown in Africa and the Indian subcontinent. There are regional variations in the UK, northern England having the highest incidence.

Table 9.1 Main features of haemophilia.

Definition	Clotting factor deficiency
Classification	Type A—Factor VIII deficiency (most common)
	Type B—Factor IX deficiency
Pathology	X-linked inheritance—Males affected
	—Females carriers
Orthopaedic problems	Joint bleeds painful and can lead to arthritis
	Soft-tissue bleeds can damage nerves
	Pseudo-tumours
Treatment	Factor replacement
	Increasing use of engineered (recombinant) forms
Complications	Human clotting factors have transmitted disease
	1200 in UK infected with HIV, none since 1986
	4800 in UK infected with hepatitis C, none since 1986
	Theoretical risk of acquiring nvCJD

Pathology

The aetiology of Paget's disease is not known, but characteristic inclusion bodies can be found in the bone cells, suggesting a viral origin. This virus may rest dormant from childhood, only being manifest later in life. Others postulate a genetic inheritance, although affected families are rare. Further research in this area is ongoing. The main feature of Paget's disease is a disordered architecture of the bone. The bones most often affected are shown in Figure 9.4.

1 Deformities are common, especially in weight-bearing bones. The tibiae become characteristically bowed.

2 Long bones become thickened, especially the cortex, and the distinction between cortex and medulla becomes lost. The trabeculae are coarsened, disordered and exaggerated.

3 The skull can become enormously thickened (Fig. 9.5), sometimes with areas of osteolysis (osteoporosis circumscripta).

4 The bones are vascular and bleed freely.

5 Fractures are common in the long bones and are typically transverse.

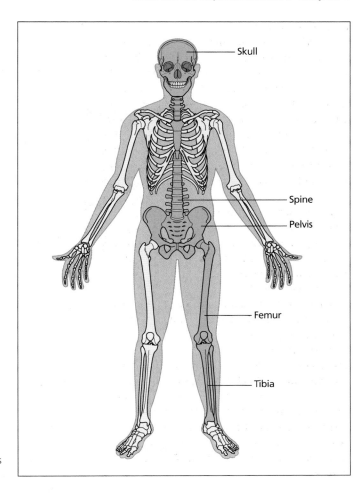

Figure **9.4** Distribution of Paget's disease.

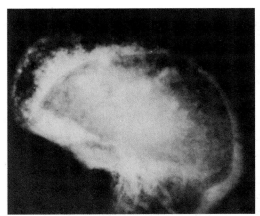

Figure 9.5 Thickening of the calvarium of the skull in Paget's disease.

6 'Pseudo' or stress fractures are also common in bones which are bowed. These are cracks with surrounding sclerosis, which may eventually progress with minimal violence to a true fracture (Fig. 9.6).
7 The vertebrae are usually affected and may be widened, with coarse trabeculae.
8 The condition may remain localized to a single bone or may be widespread.

Clinical features

Paget's original description has hardly been modified over the last 100 years. His patient was a kyphotic individual with an enlarged skull, a simian posture with wide pelvis, bowing of

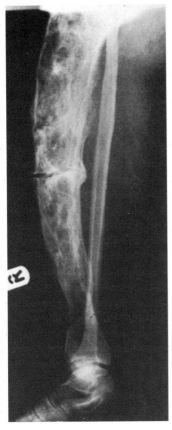

Figure 9.6 Paget's disease showing deformity of the tibia and pseudo-fractures.

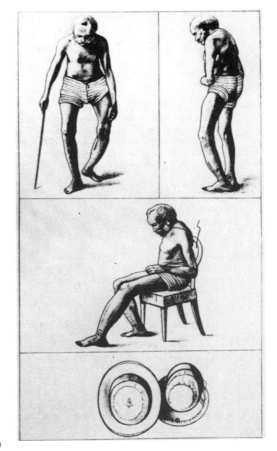

Figure 9.7 Paget's original patient.

femora and tibiae, and varus femoral necks. He developed deterioration of vision and hearing due to foraminal compression caused by thickening of the bones of the skull. He required a progressively increasing size in hats as his skull enlarged, and he eventually died from a sarcoma (Fig. 9.7).

1 Most patients remain completely symptomless and the condition is diagnosed incidentally on an X-ray.

2 In symptomatic individuals, bone pain is a relatively common presentation. It can affect any bone, particularly the tibia, and it can become disabling. Headache is a rare feature of Paget's disease of the skull.

3 Some patients complain of deformity of a long bone, usually either the tibia or femur. The radius may also become bowed, but rarely the ulna, and this may result in restriction of pronation and supination of the forearm.

4 Many patients present with one of the complications (see below), particularly a pathological fracture.

Complications

1 Pathological fractures are common and sometimes originate as a pseudo-fracture. A sudden increase in pain in the limb is usually representative of either a fracture or the development of a sarcoma.

2 Osteoarthritis frequently occurs in joints affected by Paget's disease, especially the hip. It can be difficult to distinguish the pain of arthritis from that of the Paget's disease. Joint replacement surgery can be difficult and dangerous due to bleeding.

3 Sarcomatous change occurs in less than 1% of patients, but is invariably highly malignant and is rapidly fatal. It may be an osteo-, chondro- or fibro-sarcoma. It is usually metaphyseal but may occur in the skull or vertebrae.

4 Paraplegia is rare, but may occur due to collapse of a vertebra or to vascular changes affecting the spinal cord.

5 Compression of cranial nerves leading to deafness or visual disturbances.

Diagnosis

1 Clinical and X-ray appearances.
2 Raised alkaline phosphatase.
3 Biopsy is rarely necessary unless a sarcoma is suspected.
4 Bone scan using Tc-labelled diphosphonate will usually detect the disease before it becomes visible on X-ray.

The main differential diagnosis is prostatic metastases in bone, which are similarly sclerotic and patchy.

Management

The treatment of bone pain has been made possible by the development of bisphosphonates. Calcitonin, a drug produced by the thyroid gland, is now rarely used.

Bisphosphonates reduce bone resorption by inhibiting osteoclasts which ordinarily resorb bone. They are useful for relieving pain, but their long-term effect on the bone is unknown and they can cause flu-like side effects. Disodium etidronate (EHDP; Didronel) is a first-generation bisphosphonate, is available for general use and is given orally. More recently, pamidronate, given by injection weekly for several weeks, has been used; it is a second-generation bisphosphonate whose effect may last for years. Risedronate is the most recent addition; given as a tablet it has been extensively trialled in the USA and may have lasting effects.

Apart from pain relief, treatment is usually directed to the management of fractures, although there is some evidence that deformity may be preventable. Fractures, particularly of the femur and tibia, may not always heal readily and internal fixation is often preferred. Surgery may be difficult and dangerous because of the hardness of the bone and the risk of haemorrhage. Sarcomata are generally resistant to any treatment and this can only be palliative.

Chapter 10

Inflammatory conditions

Inflammatory conditions form a heterogeneous group in which the common factor is inflammation affecting synovial membranes of joints and tendon sheaths, bursae and entheses (ligamentous insertions).

Aetiology

There have been many theories about the aetiology of these conditions, including chronic or acute infection, stress, hypersensitivity, or disturbances of collagen metabolism.

There is a clear genetic predisposition, although the mechanisms by which the genotype and the environment interact are not yet understood. Infection, with either bacteria, mycoplasmas or viruses, as yet not definitely identified, remains a possibility. These various factors perhaps initiate a sequence of synovial and articular cartilage changes, in turn mediated by lysosomal enzymes and continued by secondary immunological phenomena, including autoimmunity.

Certainly, immunological disturbances can readily be demonstrated and many humoral antibodies have been identified in this group of conditions.

Lecture Notes: Orthopaedics and Fractures, 4e.
By T Duckworth and CM Blundell. Published 2010 by Blackwell Publishing.

Pathology

The synovial membrane appears to be the target organ and is usually found to be chronically inflamed, with thickening and increased vascularity of the synovium, which forms fronds and villi.

1 There is an infiltration of vascular synovium around the periphery of the articular cartilage, forming a dull red pannus, which appears to destroy the cartilage from the edges.

2 Ligaments become softened and the joint becomes lax, particularly if there is a considerable effusion.

3 Bone erosion may lead to subarticular cysts and in severe cases ankylosis may occur.

Microscopically, the synovium is infiltrated by masses of lymphocytes and, to a lesser extent, polymorphs, and there are areas of 'fibrinoid' necrosis with granulation tissue and repair fibrosis.

Many tissues other than synovium are affected, but not all collagenous tissues suffer. In some of the inflammatory rheumatic conditions, lesions can be found in skin, lungs, abdominal viscera, muscles, heart and blood vessels, and the nervous system. The skin may be thin and loses its elasticity, and so-called 'rheumatoid nodules' are frequent.

Clinical features

Inflammatory arthritis may present acutely, acutely on chronic or chronically. These terms are subjective and have no strict diagnostic criteria, although an acute arthritis is traditionally deemed to have been present for less than 6 weeks.

The typical characteristics of joint inflammation are shown in Table 10.1.

Although the focus often is on the musculoskeletal features of inflammatory arthritis, it is important to appreciate that the majority of the conditions associated with inflammatory arthritis have systemic features and therefore, a full history should be obtained. In particular, the following should be carefully ascertained, as they will help in establishing the differential diagnosis (Table 10.2):

1 Pattern of joint involvement
2 Spinal involvement
3 Pre-existing connective tissue disease (CTD)
4 Evidence of recent infection, in particular streptococcal infection, infectious gastroenteritis and sexually-acquired infection
5 History of established inflammatory bowel disease (IBD) or symptoms suggestive of IBD—diarrhoea, rectal bleeding, rectal mucus, abdominal pain, weight loss
6 Psoriasis or first-degree family history of psoriasis
7 Ocular inflammation
8 Family history of inflammatory arthritis or CTD
9 Constitutional symptoms (fever, weight loss, night sweats)
10 History of malignancy
11 Neurological symptoms, in particular bladder and bowel dysfunction
12 Extremes of age (<16, >65).

Investigations

Blood tests

Often a barrage of investigations is required to establish the correct diagnosis. Most of these investigations require rheumatology specialist interpretation. The following are the key investigations that will assist the non-rheumatologist in an initial assessment (Table 10.3).

Full blood count

Joint inflammation may frequently produce an anaemia of chronic disease and a thrombocytosis. This gives some measure of chronicity. Several connective tissue diseases are associated with leucopenia, neutropenia, lymphopenia or thrombocytopenia.

Table 10.1 Characteristics of joint inflammation.

Pain	On joint movement
Swelling	Joint or periarticular
Heat	Especially larger superficial joints: knee, elbow, ankle, etc
Redness	Of overlying skin
Loss of function	Restricted motion and instability
Morning stiffness	Lasting more than for the first 30 min
Inactivity stiffness	Particularly in the late afternoon

Table 10.2 Important history features.

- Joints involved
- Spinal involvement
- Other connective tissue disease
- Recent infection
- Inflammatory bowel disease
- Skin disease
- Eye disease
- Family history
- Systemic symptoms
- Malignancy
- Neurological symptoms

Table 10.3 Blood tests for joint inflammation.

FBC	Routinely
ESR	Routinely
CRP	Routinely
U&E	Routinely
Bone biochemistry	Calcium, alkaline phosphatase, vitamin D
Blood cultures	If infection suspected
CPK	If myopathy
Immunoglobulins	Bence Jones protein
Bacterial and viral titres	If systemic illness
Uric acid	Not diagnostic
Ferritin	Haemochromatosis
Autoantibodies	Not specific or sensitive

Erythrocyte sedimentation rate

The erythrocyte sedimentation rate (ESR) is useful as a non-specific indicator of inflammation. It normally increases with age and will usually be elevated in the presence of anaemia.

C-reactive protein

The C-reactive protein (CRP) is an acute-phase protein produced by the liver and is again a non-specific indicator of inflammation. It is very sensitive to change and will reflect improvement or deterioration more responsively then the ESR.

The ESR and CRP are particularly useful in patients with few clinical signs; however, the following should be considered when interpreting acute phase markers:

1 An elevated ESR may be seen in patients without inflammatory disease

2 Most patients with inflammatory arthritis will have a raised ESR or CRP, although normal results do not exclude inflammation

3 A single inflamed large joint will affect the ESR and CRP to a far greater degree than 10 inflamed small (e.g. metacarpophalangeal [MCP]) joints, and therefore the ESR and CRP are not always indicative of severity

4 A raised ESR and normal CRP may be suggestive of a connective tissue disorder, e.g. lupus.

Routine biochemistry

A routine biochemical screen should be carried out to assess the degree of systemic involvement in these multi-system conditions. Primary renal and liver pathology may present with arthralgia and myalgia. Thyroid dysfunction may also present with musculoskeletal symptoms and should be considered and if appropriate excluded. Most of the drugs used to treat inflammatory arthritis can affect major organ function, hence baseline levels should be obtained prior to starting treatment.

Bone biochemistry

Calcium, alkaline phosphatase (usually included with liver function tests [LFTs]) and vitamin D levels are useful in more non-specific musculoskeletal pain. Hypovitaminosis D is increasingly being recognized and diagnosed in elderly populations.

Blood cultures

If septic arthritis is suspected blood cultures are mandatory.

Creatinine phosphokinase

A metabolic or inflammatory myopathy may present with symptoms of inflammatory arthritis. A raised creatinine phosphokinase (CPK) is associated with exercise and elevated levels must be considered in the light of a patient's exercise history.

Immunoglobulins (urine for Bence Jones protein)

Multiple myeloma may present with features of inflammatory arthritis. A polyclonal increase in immunoglobulins is invariably seen in inflammatory arthritis.

Bacterial and viral titres

Reactive arthritis is common. If there is a history of infection then objective evidence of recent infection is useful.

Uric acid

Uric acid levels have poor sensitivity and specificity for gout, and therefore neither confirm nor exclude the diagnosis. However, if gout is suspected, serum uric acid level may help with treatment and its monitoring.

Ferritin

Haemochromatosis is increasingly being recognized and may present with acute arthritis related to calcium pyrophosphate crystals (pseudogout). Untreated haemochromatosis is associated with systemic complications, including diabetes, and hepatic and cardiac dysfunction, and has an autosomal recessive inheritance pattern. Its detection is therefore important for the patient and his/her family.

Autoantibody profile

Autoantibodies typically have poor specificity and/or sensitivity and therefore there are many patients who will have false-negative or -positive results. The diagnosis of inflammatory arthritis or connective tissue disease is a clinical one, the autoantibodies only becoming important in a patient with an appropriate history and examination. Even then, a patient with a definite clinical diagnosis may have negative autoantibody tests.

Radiology

A summary of imaging modalities used in investigating and monitoring inflammatory conditions is shown in Table 10.4.

Standard musculoskeletal X-rays have traditionally been the first-line investigation for a patient with suspected inflammatory arthritis. With the advent of alternative imaging techniques, especially ultrasound and magnetic resonance imaging (MRI), this may not remain the case.

Images may be taken in order to exclude serious pathology which may mimic inflammatory arthritis, e.g. infection, tumour or fracture. They also are used to assess the 'health' of the joint in question and the degree of joint inflammation or damage.

Table 10.4 Images used in inflammatory joint disease.

Plain X-rays	Routine
Ultrasound	Soft tissues
MRI	Bone and soft tissues
Bone scintigraphy	Non-specific, good for localizing site
CT	Not widely used
DEXA scan	For osteoporosis

Sometimes the differing radiological features of inflammatory arthritis help to establish a diagnosis (Fig. 10.1). Patients and doctors are often reassured by images of the joint or soft tissues in question.

MRI and ultrasound will answer most of these questions and will frequently provide far more information than is available on plain X-ray. However, until MRI and ultrasound are widely available, traditional X-rays remain the first-line investigation.

Ultrasound

Ultrasound is increasingly used in the management of patients with inflammatory arthritis, to establish a diagnosis, to direct treatment and to monitor response to treatment. This is increasingly useful in the assessment and monitoring of drug treatment. Ultrasound is particularly useful in assessing inflammation in other synovial-lined structures, e.g. bursae and tendon sheaths.

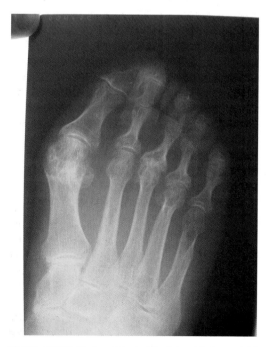

Figure 10.1 Typical radiological features of rheumatoid arthritis.

Magnetic resonance imaging

MRI is useful to establish the extent of synovitis and the involvement of soft-tissue structures, e.g. tendons, entheses, bursae, capsules and muscles. It is also very helpful if tumour or infection is being considered and the location of pathology is known. Like ultrasound, MRI is far more sensitive for articular cartilage and bone damage than X-ray.

Isotope bone scanning

Bone scintigraphy (with an injection of Technetium[99]) is useful if it is uncertain where the pathology (inflammation, tumour or infection) is located and the potential area concerned is too large to allow straightforward MRI examination, e.g. in patients with pelvic pain, or if multifocal inflammation, tumour or infection is suspected. Bone scintigraphy is also helpful in excluding significant musculoskeletal inflammation in patients without clear symptoms or signs.

Computed tomography

Musculoskeletal CTs are rarely helpful in the assessment of patients with inflammatory arthritis.

Dual energy X-ray absorptiometry

Osteoporosis is a complication of arthritis and its treatment, especially systemic steroids. There are several ways in which bone density can be assessed, although the most validated method in terms of establishing fracture risk is DEXA.

Synovial fluid analysis

Appearance

Normal synovial fluid has a very pale yellow hue, is transparent and has a normal viscosity, which can only be appreciated with experience. Progressive levels of inflammation are associated with increasing levels of cellularity with increasing turbidity (increasingly yellow with loss of clarity) and loss of normal viscosity. Inflammatory arthritis is usually associated with a deeper yellow colour and some clarity.

Microbiological analysis

Microbiological analysis is essential if septic arthritis is considered possible. Synovial fluid should be obtained prior to giving antibiotics and be followed by intravenous antibiotics to cover the likely pathogens until culture results are available.

Histological analysis

Histological analysis of synovial fluid can be extremely helpful in specialist hands.

Crystal analysis

The presence of monosodium urate and calcium pyrophosphate crystals in synovial fluid is diagnostic for gout and pseudo-gout respectively. Urate crystals are usually very obvious and their absence almost certainly means the diagnosis is not gout. Calcium pyrophosphate crystals are very difficult to see even in experienced hands.

Medical management of inflammatory arthritis

Controlling synovitis

The underlying principle of managing inflammatory arthritis is that joint inflammation causes irreversible joint damage, which causes disability and handicap. The control of joint inflammation is imperative in order to preserve joint function. Drugs that have been shown to control synovitis and prevent or attenuate joint inflammation and subsequent damage fall into three categories:

1 Disease modifying anti-rheumatic drugs (DMARDs)
2 Biological therapies
3 Steroids.

Non-steroidal anti-inflammatory drugs (NSAIDs) are tremendously useful at reducing pain, swelling and stiffness, but do not influence the underlying inflammatory process in terms of preventing or reducing joint damage and are only used for symptom control.

Disease-modifying anti-rheumatic drugs
The most commonly used drugs in current practice are methotrexate, leflunomide and sulfasalazine. They all broadly share the same characteristics:

1 Reduce synovitis and therefore improve symptoms, improve function and reduce the likelihood of permanent joint damage
2 Slow acting, may take up to 3–6 months to have their full effect
3 Effective in about 70% of patients
4 Side effect profile requires the regular monitoring of blood tests (FBC, U&E, LFT)
5 May be used alone or in combination
6 Treatment is escalated in terms of dose and combinations until control of synovitis is achieved
7 Full remission of arthritis is unlikely
8 Do not have a negative effect on wound healing and do not increase the risk of post-operative infection. They can be safely used peri-operatively.

Biological therapies
Biological therapies are 'designer' drugs aimed at blocking particular components of the inflammatory cascade. The only biological therapies widely used in clinical practice are drugs that reduce or block tumour necrosis factor (TNF) activity. Drugs currently available are infliximab, etanercept and adalumimab. They all share the same characteristics:

1 Work quickly (within 4 weeks)
2 Given by injection (infliximab as IV injection, etanercept and adalumimab as subcutaneous injection)
3 Research suggests that they are effective in 70% of patients, although clinical observations suggest a better response rate
4 More effective if co-prescribed with methotrexate
5 Require monitoring with regular blood tests
6 Main side effect is an increased risk of serious and non-serious infection, in particular tuberculosis.

In the UK, because of their cost, they are currently rationed for use when conventional

Table 10.5 DMARDs contrasted with biological therapies.

DMARDS	Biological therapies
Long to act (3–6 months)	Quick to act (<4 weeks)
Effective in 70%	Effective in >70%
Orally available	Intravenous only usage
Unlikely to be curative	Can be curative
Safe for surgery	Stop 2 weeks prior to surgery

DMARDs have failed, although they are more widely available in the USA (Table 10.5).

Current evidence suggests that they should be increasingly considered as first-line treatment with methotrexate. Complete remission seems to be achievable in some patients. They should be withdrawn 2 weeks before elective surgery and restarted 2 weeks post-operatively, assuming there are no signs of post-operative infection.

Steroids
Steroids can be given as injections (intra-articular, -venous, -muscular) or in oral form.

Injectable steroids have a rapid onset of action and are widely used, particularly intra-articular steroids. In the context of mono- (single joint) or oligo- (fewer than four joints) arthritis, an intra-articular steroid injection can be extremely effective.

Oral steroids have been used in rheumatological practice for many years. They are very effective at reducing inflammation, but unfortunately their long-term use is limited by dose-dependent side effects. Consequently they are not used long-term at doses greater than 5–7.5 mg daily. With the advent of anti-TNF treatments, the use of long-term oral steroids will probably decrease.

Other aspects of management
In addition to controlling synovitis, the medical care of patients with inflammatory arthritis includes a number of additional aspects: prevention of disease- or treatment-associated side effects, e.g. preserving bone health, proactively managing cardiovascular risk factors. In addition there should be close liaison with surgeons to ensure that referrals are made appropriately and expeditiously.

Table 10.6 Non-infectious inflammatory arthritis.

Descriptive term	Associated conditions	Notes
Seropositive arthritis	Rheumatoid arthritis (RA)	RA is not always seropositive
Monoarthritis	Psoriasis	Seronegative arthritides are frequently
Oligoarthritis (fewer	Inflammatory bowel disease	associated with characteristic
than four joints	Reactive arthritis	extra-articular features, e.g. uveitis,
affected)		genitourinary symptoms, skin rashes
Spondyloarthropathy	Ankylosing spondylitis	Inflammatory arthritis involving the sacroiliac
	Psoriasis	joints and spine in addition to peripheral
	Inflammatory bowel disease	joints. All seronegative arthropathies are
	Reactive arthritis	associated with HLAB27
Crystal arthropathy	Gout	Confirmation of crystals in synovial fluid is
	Pseudo-gout	the gold standard for diagnosis
Connective tissue diseases	Systemic lupus	Arthritis is only feature of these multi-system
	Scleroderma	illnesses but this highlights the importance
Systemic vasculitis	Wegener's granulomatosis	of taking a full history when presented
	Polyarteritis nodosa	with an acute arthritis
Multi-system illness	Sarcoidosis	

(Left margin label spanning rows: Seronegative arthritis)

Multi-disciplinary team (MDT) care is required as patients with inflammatory arthritis require support from the doctors of a range of disciplines, as well as specialist nurses, physiotherapists, occupational therapists, podiatrists, orthotists and psychologists.

Inflamed joints undergo the same functional deterioration as injured joints and therefore rehabilitation is vital to restoring normal joint function. With the exception of an acutely inflamed joint, when pain rather than any evidence that exercise induces damage is the limiting factor, patients with inflammatory arthritis should be encouraged to rehabilitate proactively. The same generic rehabilitation principles apply to a previously inflamed joint as would apply to an injured joint.

Aspects of non-infectious inflammatory arthritis are summarized in Table 10.6.

Rheumatoid arthritis

Rheumatoid arthritis (RA) is a common disease, affecting 1% of the UK population, usually occurring in middle age and in women more than men. It usually presents with slowly increasing stiffness and aching in the small peripheral joints, particularly of the hands, and may progress to cause severe incapacity and deformity.

Clinical features

The mode of presentation, the joints affected, and the subsequent progress are very variable.

The disease may begin in one or several joints and may progress rapidly with almost continual acute inflammation in the joints, or it may begin insidiously with morning stiffness only, perhaps progressing in semi-acute exacerbations, each involving more and more joints. Occasionally, the first manifestation of the disease may be a carpal tunnel syndrome or isolated tenosynovitis. The hands, wrists and knees are usually involved, but most joints can be affected, including those of the spine.

There is often weight loss, weakness and loss of appetite, and, rarely, there may be mild fever during the acute attacks.

Eventually, the joints become obviously inflamed, swollen with fluid and synovial thickening, restricted in movement and often with ligamentous laxity, allowing deformities such as the characteristic ulnar deviation of the fingers (Fig. 10.2) to develop.

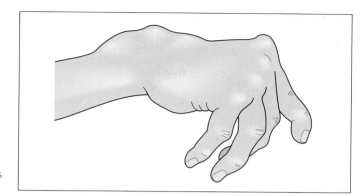

Figure 10.2 Rheumatoid arthritis affecting the hand.

The joints are tender and feel 'boggy', and there may be much muscle spasm. Tendon sheaths also swell, particularly in the hand, and cause pain on finger movements. Occasionally, the infiltrated tendons rupture, producing secondary deformities and loss of function. Destruction of joint surfaces may also contribute to deformity in late cases.

Remissions occur, usually temporarily, but occasionally the disease appears to burn out. The deformities are, of course, permanent. Secondary osteoarthritic changes are very common.

RA is a multisystem disease and is associated with complications that can affect all the major organs. As a result it is associated with increased mortality. This seems to be largely attributable to increased cardiovascular mortality, hence there is an increasing appreciation of the importance of managing cardiovascular risk factors as is the case for diabetics.

Radiological changes

The earliest change is usually a diffuse porosis around the joint due to the effects of cytokines, with increased vascularity. Later, the joint space may become narrowed and destruction of the joint surface may be obvious (Fig. 10.3). Subluxation and dislocation are common and occasionally ankylosis (spontaneous fusion) occurs.

Diagnosis

The diagnosis is usually made on clinical grounds, but early or monoarticular cases may be difficult

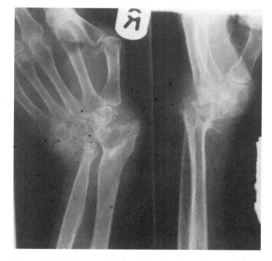

Figure 10.3 Rheumatoid arthritis affecting the wrist joint.

to diagnose. The ESR is usually raised and sometimes the white cell count is increased.

Agglutination tests, such as the sheep cell and latex tests, eventually become positive in at least 70% of cases. They are not often helpful in diagnosis, but tend to relate to severity.

Synovial biopsy may be useful in excluding infective conditions such as tuberculosis.

Management

Medical

During the acute stages, rest and a helpful environment appear desirable, but their effects are uncertain. Bed rest may be needed, but contrastingly retaining mobility is important. Local measures include splinting painful joints followed by passive exercises when the pain becomes less, with long-term active exercises to maintain mobility. Wax baths and hydrotherapy all have a place.

Systemic therapy
This is essentially the management of a polyarthropathy, as described above.

Surgery
Surgery has gradually offered more and more to the rheumatoid patient but careful selection of patients is essential. The surgical options are summarized in Box 10.1.

1 **Synovectomy**, i.e. removing the diseased synovium, can give excellent relief of pain, but there is conflicting evidence as to whether it slows down joint destruction. The knees and the joints of the fingers are best suited to this procedure. The synovium regrows in 3–4 weeks, but the rheumatoid process appears to be delayed, sometimes for several years. Synovectomy of tendon sheaths may prevent tendon rupture.

2 **Repair of ruptured tendons and capsular procedures** may restore active movement to the fingers.

3 **Joint fusion**. Certain joints such as the wrist benefit from fusion, but for most joints arthroplasty is more likely to give good function. Fusion of adjacent vertebrae may be necessary in the cervical spine when subluxation threatens cord damage.

4 **Arthroplasty**. A wide range of procedures is available, using the same prostheses as those for osteoarthritis. The results are often better than with osteoarthritis because the functional demands of the patient are less, but the risk of sepsis, particularly in patients on steroids, is considerable. Surgery is usually performed when the disease is well controlled by systemic therapy.

Box 10.1 Surgery in rheumatoid arthritis.

- Synovectomy
- Tendon repair
- Arthrodesis
- Arthroplasty

Social and supportive measures
These are all important in maintaining morale and independence. The patient's work may need to be modified, and appliances and home circumstances designed to cope with his/her disability. Nevertheless, many patients do not reach this degree of severity and of those who do, most remain surprisingly independent.

Juvenile chronic arthritis

The disease in children is the equivalent of the adult condition and is characterized by its systemic effects. It is much less common than the adult form.

The term *juvenile chronic arthritis* includes Still's disease and a number of less well-defined conditions, some of which may be monoarticular or may have minimal joint involvement—so-called *pauciarticular*.

Clinical features
The onset is often insidious, but may be acute. Fever, lymph gland involvement and anaemia are usually present in addition to the joint pains and stiffness. Uveitis occasionally occurs.

The main joints affected are the knees, ankles, wrists and occasionally the spine. The degree of pain varies, children occasionally presenting with chronically swollen joints which are painless and functioning normally.

Deformities occur, as in the adult form, and there is a more marked tendency to ankylosis, especially in the cervical spine. Epiphyseal growth may be disturbed.

Radiological features
As in the adult rheumatoid, these may not be striking in the early stages. The changes are essentially the same, although much less marked. The carpus is usually affected and fusion of the wrist may occur.

Diagnosis
The ESR is usually raised, but serological tests are usually negative, except in the pauciarticular form. Pericarditis and a history of preceding strep-

tococcal infection favours the diagnosis of rheumatic fever, although this is now rare in the UK. In the monoarticular case, the distinction is usually from osteomyelitis or suppurative arthritis.

Treatment

The same local and general measures are needed as in the adult. Physiotherapy is important in maintaining joint movements, particularly when the disease is beginning to settle. Surgery is rarely needed, and synovectomy, although occasionally used, is usually followed by a very long period of rehabilitation. After the disease has subsided, surgery may be helpful in restoring joint movement by dividing tight contractures, adhesions, etc. Occasionally, osteotomies may be necessary to correct severe deformities.

Prognosis

The outlook is good: 60–75% of patients recover fully, although this may take several years. A few patients become severely disabled and death may occur from visceral involvement.

Seronegative arthritides

A range of conditions may be considered under this heading. Management depends on the nature of the joint involvement, with each condition having its own characteristics. Dactylitis, the uniform sausage-like swelling of a digit, is diagnostic of seronegative arthritides. Enthesitis is another typical feature and may be overlooked as a mechanical tendinopathy unless an inflammatory cause is considered.

Polymyalgia rheumatica

This is a form of rheumatic disease usually occurring in patients over the age of 60. It is rare under 50 years of age. It affects women more than men and is characterized by aching pain and stiffness in the muscles of the neck, shoulder girdle and occasionally in the back and pelvic girdle. In approximately 20% of cases it is associated with arteritis of the cranial vessels and sudden blindness due to occlusion of the retinal artery is a constant risk.

Diagnosis

This is essentially clinical, but the ESR is usually considerably raised and biopsy of the temporal artery may reveal the associated arteritis.

Treatment

High doses of steroids, e.g. 50–60 mg of prednisolone per day, are recommended for cranial arteritis, but lower doses, i.e. less than 20 mg per day are adequate for polymyalgia rheumatica. The disease usually subsides over a period of months or years.

Ankylosing spondylitis

This is a well-defined condition. The histocompatibility antigen HLA-B27 is detectable in about 90% of patients with the disease. This has also been found in associated conditions such as anterior uveitis and Reiter's syndrome.

Clinical features

The disease, which is essentially an enthesitis, tends to affect young adults—males more than females. It usually starts with pain and stiffness in the lumbar region and over a period of months or years this gradually extends to involve the whole spine and the manubriosternal joints.

The characteristic feature is ossification of the ligaments of the spine and the intervertebral discs, so that the spine is converted into a solid rod, usually with a gradually increasing kyphos (bamboo spine; Fig. 10.4). In severe cases the patient may not be able to raise his/her head to see forwards. Other joints may be involved, particularly the larger joints, with rheumatoid-like symptoms and signs, and a tendency to severe stiffness. The sacroiliac joints are affected as a necessary prerequisite for the diagnosis and the radiological appearances of irregularity and marginal sclerosis with eventual fusion are very characteristic. Plantar fasciitis, Achilles tendinitis and tenderness over bony prominences are common.

Fibrosis of the lungs and aortitis also occur and iridocyclitis is an occasional accompaniment. The ESR is usually, but not always, raised. Tests for rheumatoid factor are negative.

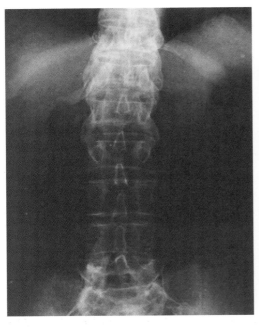 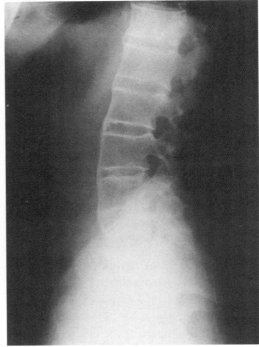

Figure 10.4 Ankylosing spondylitis producing intervertebral fusions.

Treatment

It is rarely possible to influence the pathological course of this condition. Phenylbutazone is useful in relieving painful joint symptoms and backache, but because of its toxicity it should only be considered if other NSAIDs have failed. In the UK, it is now licensed only for hospital use for this condition.

Physiotherapy, particularly exercises to maintain joint movement, may be helpful in early cases, and a period of rest in a corrective plaster shell may be needed if deformity is progressing quickly. Severely deformed patients may require a corrective osteotomy of the spine. The disease usually progresses slowly, but its activity may eventually lessen, leaving the patient with residual problems which may need such measures as joint replacement.

Acute synovitis (monoarthritis or the 'acute painful joint')

Patients frequently present with a swollen painful joint, with an obvious effusion and often with syn-

ovial thickening. The knee is the most commonly affected. Many of these represent the earliest manifestation of rheumatoid disease, but investigations should be carried out with the following possibilities in mind:

1 Rheumatoid arthritis
2 Reiter's syndrome (or septic arthritis due to gonococcus)
3 Psoriasis (which produces an arthropathy very similar to rheumatoid arthritis)
4 Ulcerative colitis
5 Ankylosing spondylitis
6 Tuberculosis
7 Gout.

Reiter's syndrome

The synovitis or arthritis is associated with non-specific urethritis and conjunctivitis. The disease is either sexually transmitted or associated with bacillary dysentery.

Clinical features

The arthritis may be acute or of gradual onset, and may be widespread or monoarticular. The ophthalmic symptoms and urethritis may occur separately. Plantar fasciitis and Achilles tendinitis may be a feature. The arthritis is usually self-limiting, but recurrence is common. The ESR is usually raised. Rheumatoid factor tests are negative. HLA-B27 antigen is present in over 70% of cases. In the chronic case, periostitis is a common feature. Sacroiliitis occurs as in ankylosing spondylitis.

Treatment

The urethritis, which may be non-specific or related to chlamydial infection, may be treated with antibiotics, but it is difficult to eliminate. Chronic joint symptoms are treated by rest in the acute phase, with physiotherapy and anti-inflammatory drugs as necessary.

Psoriatic arthritis

About 5–10% of patients with psoriasis suffer from a polyarthritis of rheumatoid type. Usually, the small joints of the hands and feet are affected. Distal interphalangeal joints may be involved and there may be large joint, sacroiliac or spondylotic changes.

This is a seronegative arthritis; the disease may be asymmetrical with little periarticular osteoporosis and the skin lesions are characteristic.

Treatment

This is similar to that for rheumatoid arthritis, but the prognosis is usually better.

Reactive arthritis

The term reactive arthritis refers to inflammatory arthritis that has been triggered by an infection rather than infection within a joint (septic arthritis). The arthritis seems to reflect immunological cross-reactivity and usually develops within 2 weeks of the infection but may be delayed following some infections. Monoarthritis is the most common presentation. Virtually every infection has at some time been associated with a reactive arthritis. Streptococcal infections and those causing infectious gastroenteritis and genitourinary infection are most notable, although the common viral upper respiratory tract infection (URTI) is probably most often to blame. This is usually self-limiting. Chlamydia infection is often asymptomatic and a careful and sensitive history is essential. Referral to a genitourinary medicine department should be considered in all patients.

Gout

This is a metabolic disease characterized by the deposition of urates in the tissues, hyperuricaemia and, in about 10% of cases, increased excretion of uric acid in the urine. It is a common disease, affecting men in 95% of cases and post-menopausal women. The arthritis usually affects the distal joints of the hands and feet, and the knees. It particularly (and characteristically) affects the metatarsophalangeal joints of the great toes, though these are by no means always involved.

Clinical features

The disease is chronic, but characterized by acute attacks in which the affected joints, usually single, become severely painful, swollen, often red and impossible to move. This usually settles spontaneously in less than 3 weeks. The joint may be gradually damaged by repeated attacks. Other features include the formation of gouty tophi—collections of urate crystals in the soft tissues, especially in the ear lobes, hands and feet.

Over the years, the condition gradually becomes more generalized. Any form of trauma, including surgery, may precipitate an attack, as may alcohol, certain antibiotics and purine-rich foods, such as liver. Renal complications such as stone formation are well-recognized and, rarely, renal failure may lead to deterioration and death.

Investigations

The X-ray appearance may be typical, with well-demarcated, rounded erosions close to the joint margins, usually in the hands. Joint destruction may be seen later.

The most useful investigation is the serum uric acid, which is usually well above normal, although occasionally isolated readings may be within normal limits.

Treatment

Two drugs are useful for treating the acute attack:

1 Colchicine, which is very specific and may be used as a therapeutic test. It is, however, toxic and unpleasant to take

2 NSAIDs, such as indometacin or diclofenac, are usually effective.

Many patients are also treated with a drug such as allopurinol which lowers the serum uric acid in the anticipation of preventing further attacks.

Nevertheless, acute attacks may be precipitated by allopurinol or probenecid if given without NSAID cover.

Pseudo-gout

This is a condition which is, in some respects, similar to gout, but is usually less acute, and the crystals deposited in the affected joint are of calcium pyrophosphate rather than uric acid. A common feature is calcification of the menisci of the knees, although this is rather non-specific. There is usually evidence of osteoarthritis. No specific treatment is known, but NSAIDs are usually helpful in relieving symptoms.

Chapter 11

Degenerative conditions

Degenerative conditions are those in which the tissues in question gradually stop functioning. The causes are often poorly understood. The conditions are considered as those affecting articular cartilage and those affecting tissues predominantly made of collagen.

Degenerative conditions of articular cartilage

Degenerative changes commonly occur in hyaline articular cartilage, culminating in the fully developed condition of osteoarthritis, often called osteoarthrosis because it is essentially a non-inflammatory condition.

The precise point at which degeneration can be called true osteoarthritis is difficult to establish. The earliest change in the cartilage, i.e. the development of minute splits and softening of the surface, may not always progress to fully-established arthritis.

Osteoarthritis

This is a disease of synovial joints in which the articular cartilage becomes split, fissured and softened, and gradually resorbs, sometimes down to

Lecture Notes: Orthopaedics and Fractures, 4e.
By T Duckworth and CM Blundell. Published 2010 by Blackwell Publishing.

underlying bone. The subchondral bone then becomes thickened and hard, known as eburnated, and there is proliferation of new bone around the edges of the articular surface, leading to the formation of spurs of bone called osteophytes. Secondary changes occur in the capsule and ligaments, and the joint becomes stiffened and painful.

Pathology
The changes appear to begin in articular cartilage with softening and splitting known as fibrillation. Research is proceeding vigorously into the causation of the condition. Attempts are being made to answer the following two questions:

1 Is the disease primarily one of cartilage?
2 Are the changes preceded by changes in the underlying bone?

Primary cartilage disease
Most of the indications point in this direction, and there are two main possibilities:

1 The changes may be essentially biochemical; or
2 The changes may be essentially mechanical.

It may well be that mechanical changes lead to biochemical changes or indeed biochemical changes may lead onto mechanical changes. It seems likely that there is an interplay of the two processes.

BIOCHEMICAL
1 The collagen may be affected under the influence of matrix metalloproteinases. These enzymes

and others perhaps responsible for collagen break-down are regulated by a group of compounds termed TIMPS (tissue inhibitors of metalloprotein-ases). Regulation of these proteins may hold the key as to the collagen changes seen in osteoarthritis and this is being actively investigated.

2 The proteoglycan matrix may be abnormal. Changes in proteoglycan ratios can be demonstrated in osteoarthritic cartilage and these may affect water-binding capacity and hence mechanical strength. Certain hormones are known to affect proteoglycan metabolism, e.g. osteoarthritis is particularly prone to occur in acromegalic patients.

MECHANICAL

The collagen might wear or disrupt, allowing proteoglycan matrix to leak out. This could occur as a result of either:

1 Fatigue failure, perhaps due to defective lubrication.

2 Abrasive wear—caused by high spots or incongruities in the joint.

The importance of synovial fluid in maintaining cartilage requires further study. Some incongruity between the joint surfaces is necessary for fluid circulation.

Underlying bone changes

1 Changes in bone density can often be demonstrated in osteoarthritic joints.

2 The bone often shows marked haemodynamic changes, particularly affecting the venous circulation.

3 The bony architecture is often abnormal as a result of previous trauma or disease.

4 The bone often shows trabecular fractures and cysts, although usually late in the condition.

Pathogenesis

Osteoarthritis is classified as either primary (no known underlying cause) or secondary (to a known cause). Secondary causes of osteoarthritis include:

1 Fractures (especially intra-articular injuries) (see Chapter 6)

2 Joint infection

3 Inflammatory joint disease

4 Congenital joint abnormalities

> **Box 11.1** Symptoms of osteoarthritis.
>
> - Stiffness
> - Swelling
> - Deformity

---

5 Joint instability

6 Cartilage damage

7 Obesity.

Weight-bearing joints, especially the hip and the knee, are most frequently affected. Osteoarthritis, once established, is usually a progressive disorder. Rarely, a patient presents with widespread osteoarthritic changes in many joints. This is sometimes an inherited condition.

Clinical features (see also Box 11.1)

(see Part 2 for details of the particular joints)

1 **Pain** is the usual presenting feature—usually slowly increasing in severity as the joint stiffens. Morning pain may indicate a more inflammatory component (see Chapter 10). The pain is usually exacerbated by exercise, but the joint often feels stiff after rest. Pain-disturbed sleep is an important index of severity.

2 **Stiffness** may make tasks such as putting on socks difficult, but is not usually in itself a major cause of complaint.

3 **Swelling** of the joint results from over-production or under-absorption of synovial fluid. Bony swelling may result from osteophyte formation.

4 **Deformity** tends to develop as a result of more severe destruction of the underlying bone surface, especially at the knee and the ankle. Deformity also results from soft-tissue changes such as muscular spasm—the stronger muscle groups overcoming the weak, or from capsular and ligamentous contracture. Deformity can interfere with function, particularly gait, and affects the nearby joints which become abnormally loaded.

Physical signs (see also Box 11.2)

ON INSPECTION

1 Fixed deformities.

2 Swelling due to moderate synovial thickening and bony enlargement of the joint due to

> **Box 11.2** Physical signs of osteoarthritis.
>
> - Deformity
> - Tenderness
> - Limited movement
> - Crepitus
> - Abnormal function (e.g. limp)

osteophytes and occasional effusions during acute episodes.

ON PALPATION

1 Tenderness around the joint.
2 Swelling.

ON MOVING

1 Restriction of movements which may become almost total, although fusion does not occur.
2 Muscle spasm and pain on attempting movements beyond the 'limit'.
3 Crepitus (a 'crunching or grinding feeling') on movement.
4 Abnormalities of gait or upper limb function.

Radiological signs

1 Narrowing of the joint space—the most important sign.
2 Osteophyte formation around the edges of the joint.
3 Sclerosis in the subchondral bone.
4 Cysts in the subchondral bone.

Management

Non-operative

The condition is a slowly progressive and painful one, and most patients can be managed conservatively for many years.

1 Analgesics are usually the mainstay of treatment. Anti-inflammatory analgesics are of less help in osteoarthritis than in rheumatoid arthritis.
2 Protection of the joint, e.g. the patient may benefit by losing weight, and a stick, splint or other support may be helpful.
3 Change of lifestyle, such as a more sedentary job.

4 Physiotherapy, i.e. intermittent heat treatment or short-wave diathermy, with supervised exercises to maintain movements.

Surgical

Surgery may be needed, particularly when sleep is disturbed or quality of life has been substantially reduced. There are various surgical possibilities of varying magnitude, and each patient needs to be assessed carefully before a decision is made.

OSTEOTOMY

For certain joints in younger patients an osteotomy, usually close to the joint, e.g. through the upper tibia for the knee, can relieve pain dramatically. It is especially effective when part of the joint remains uninvolved and re-alignment changes the loading characteristics. It is usually reserved for joints with a reasonable range of movement.

ARTHRODESIS

The correct term for a joint fusion in which the bones either side of the joint are joined together permanently. This can be the most certain way of relieving pain, especially in the young person. It always causes some disability but if sound it will stand up to heavy stresses over many years. It is used particularly for small joints, such as those in the hand and foot. The nearby joints have to compensate for the loss of movement and may subsequently also degenerate.

ARTHROPLASTY

This is the official name for joint replacement, now usually carried out with artificial materials. This is the age of the arthroplasty and many artificial replacements are available for almost every joint from finger joints, through knees to intervertebral discs. The hip and knee have received most attention and very satisfactory pain relief and function can now be attained.

The goal now is to develop joints with long survival so that they may be used on younger and higher demand individuals. Attention is also now being focused on replacing joints through small incisions to encourage early return to full function with less morbidity.

ARTHROSCOPIC LAVAGE

Clearing out debris, osteophytes, cartilage fragments, etc, sometimes with partial synovectomy, can be a useful palliative procedure, and has been used especially for the knee. However, a recent placebo controlled randomized study of 180 patients questioned the benefit and the technique is being used less and less.

Many factors need to be considered in deciding which surgical treatment is best for each patient. These include age, occupation, general mobility, psychological make-up, severity of symptoms and the condition of other joints. The final decision will usually involve balancing the risks of the procedure against the likely advantages.

Degenerative conditions of collagenous tissues

This group of conditions is characterized by deterioration in the structure and strength of those tissues that contain a high proportion of collagen, i.e. tendons, joint capsules, fascia and intervertebral discs. The cause is unknown, but this type of pathology becomes more common with ageing, and in some respects has features suggesting an accelerated ageing process. Inflammation is not a major feature, but may occur as a reaction to injury or spontaneous rupture and be part of the healing process.

Several of the conditions described below may occur simultaneously or at intervals in the same patient. They seem to form part of a syndrome of degenerative conditions affecting collagenous tissues.

Each region-specific condition is dealt with in detail under the relevant region in Part 2.

Tendinopathy

Tendinopathies are a group of conditions affecting the tendons themselves and are characterized by swelling, tenderness and gradual loss of function. The collagen becomes disorganized with the constant splitting (tendinosis), inflammation (tendonitis) and subsequent healing, resulting in a tendon sometimes many times its original girth.

Gradually the tendon loses its elasticity and original length. Examples include the Achilles tendon, tibialis posterior tendon and others. Acute ruptures are excluded.

Treatment
Rest and if necessary, immobilization are often all that is needed. Sometimes a splint to off-load the tendon helps. Rarely, injections of steroid or surgery are used.

Tenosynovitis

This is a condition in which a tendon sheath becomes inflamed and often distended with fluid. The cause sometimes appears to be trauma, particularly associated with repetitive movements. It usually affects the flexor or extensor tendons of the thumb or fingers where they cross the wrist within a synovial sheath. The area is tender and movements of the tendon cause pain, often radiating to the appropriate digit and sometimes associated with crepitus. The symptoms are usually chronic, unlike those associated with suppurative tenosynovitis. Examples are De Quervain's disease and trigger fingers.

Treatment
A change of occupation may be sufficient to relieve the symptoms; otherwise a period of 2–3 weeks' immobilization in a plaster-cast, extended to prevent thumb or finger movements, is usually curative.

Intervertebral disc degeneration

The young intervertebral disc consists of a well-demarcated nucleus pulposus and annulus fibrosus. Starting in early adult life, changes occur in the matrix chemistry, with the proportions of the mucopolysaccharide constituents becoming altered in such a way that the water-binding properties are diminished. In addition, the fibrous content of the nucleus increases until in old age the disc consists almost completely of a collagen feltwork. In consequence, the disc loses its elasticity and ability to act as a shock absorber and the disc space becomes narrowed and distorted. These changes occur in everyone with age, but in some individuals the changes seem to progress more rapidly and must be regarded as pathological. In the early stages of this degenerative process, the changes may occur unevenly within the disc and considerable stresses may be set up. Such stresses, coupled with a localized weakness of the annulus, may allow nuclear material to burst through the annulus, particularly during lifting or straining—this condition is usually called disc prolapse.

Capsulitis

This is most frequently seen in the shoulder and is discussed in detail in Chapter 18. The collagen of the joint capsule may give way and become inflamed. There is sometimes deposition of calcium in the degenerate tissues. This may result from ageing or trauma, or may be idiopathic. Chronically in the shoulder it is often know as 'frozen shoulder', as it results in stiffness.

Ganglion

This presents as a cystic swelling occurring in relation to a joint or tendon sheath. Ganglia are particularly common on the dorsum of the hand and wrist and around the ankle. Small ganglia on the palmar aspect of the fingers may be very tense and can feel like a small pea.

The typical ganglion arises insidiously and may vary in size. It is often not tender, but may cause local aching. It is fluctuant and transilluminable. It is filled with a gel which is thought to be derived from synovial fluid. It is believed to arise by a protrusion of synovium or synovial fluid through a microscopic split in the capsule or fibrous sheath, the opening acting as a flap-valve. This accounts for its tendency to vary in size or to disappear, and also for the fact that it occasionally develops after trauma to the wrist or foot.

Treatment

A ganglion may be dispersed by a blow or pressure with traditional treatment being to hit it with 'the family bible'. It may also be aspirated. Recurrence is usual following these manoeuvres, and surgical removal may be necessary. The neck of the ganglion must be excised if recurrence is to be avoided.

Miscellaneous conditions

Various other conditions occur when the collagenous tissues degenerate, and these are described in Part 2. Examples are tennis elbow, golfer's elbow, Dupuytren's contracture and plantar fasciitis.

Chapter 12

Neoplastic conditions of bone and soft tissue

General principles

The definition of a neoplasm is a group of cells which continue to proliferate indefinitely in an uncontrolled fashion. The distinction between these cells and those which proliferate for a time, eventually becoming mature, is a blurred one. It is convenient to define the second group as hamartomata.

True tumours are usually sub-divided into benign and malignant but, again, the distinction is not always clear either from the histological or behavioural point of view.

Bone tumours

A classification of the commonest type of bone tumours is given below:
1 **Hamartomas**:
  - Fibrous cortical defect
  - Fibrous dysplasia
  - Simple bone cyst
2 **Benign bone tumours**:
  - Aneurysmal bone cyst
  - Enchondroma
  - Osteochondroma
  - Chondroblastoma

- Chondromyxoid fibroma
- Osteoid osteoma/osteoblastoma
- Giant cell tumour
3 **Malignant bone tumours**:
  - Osteosarcoma
  - Ewing's sarcoma
  - Chondrosarcoma
  - Spindle cell sarcomas (including fibrosarcoma., leiomyosarcoma, Malignant Fibrous Histiocytoma)
4 **Haematological malignancies**:
  - Plasmacytoma/myeloma
  - Non-Hodgkin's lymphoma
5 **Metastases to bone**: mostly from epithelial cancers, the commonest being breast, bronchus, prostate, thyroid and kidney.

Presentation

Most bone tumours present with a history of increasing bone in the affected limb, sometimes accompanied by a swelling and sometimes followed by a pathological fracture. The key investigation for any patient with non-specific pain, particularly non-mechanical pain (i.e. not related to movement) is a plain X-ray of the affected part. The radiological features that indicate a pathological process is going on in the bone which requires further investigation are shown in the Box 12.1.

The presence of any of these should lead to further investigation of the patient to identify the cause. Potential causes apart from bone tumours

Lecture Notes: Orthopaedics and Fractures, 4e.
By T Duckworth and CM Blundell. Published 2010 by Blackwell Publishing.

Box 12.1 Radiological features indicative of pathological process.

- Bone destruction
- New bone formation
- Periosteal reaction
- Soft tissue swelling

Box 12.2 Stepwise assessment of a suspected case.

- History
- Examination
- Simple tests: X-ray, bloods
- Scan: bone or CT
- MRI
- Biopsy

---

include: developmental abnormalities, infection and metabolic deficiencies.

Investigation of a patient with an abnormal area of bone

The aim of investigating the patient is to reach a diagnosis in as short a time as possible. The most likely diagnosis will often be indicated by the patient's age and the plain X-ray appearance, e.g. a lytic destructive tumour in an adolescent is likely to be a sarcoma, but in a 65-year-old it is likely to be a metastasis. Box 12.2 summarizes the investigative process.

Step 1. Take a detailed history from the patient, including past medical history (cancer) and current symptoms (e.g. a cough in a smoker may indicate lung cancer). In older patients, enquire particularly about symptoms related to tumours that are known to metastasize to bone (breast, bronchus, thyroid, kidney and prostate).

Step 2. Examine the patient, including sites of potential primary tumours (breast, bronchus, thyroid, kidney and prostate).

Step 3. Arrange simple investigations, including chest X-ray and blood tests (full blood count, erythrocyte sedimentation rate and biochemical profile as a minimum, in older patients include prostate-specific antigen and myeloma screen).

Step 4. If no diagnosis is apparent, arrange a bone scan to see if the lesion is solitary, and in patients

over the age of 35 arrange for CT chest and abdomen.

Step 5. If the lesion is solitary and no diagnosis is still apparent, arrange an MRI of the tumour and refer the patient to a tumour centre for biopsy.

Biopsy

Biopsies are usually carried out under X-ray or CT control using needles. Samples must be sent for both histology and microbiology (to rule out infection) in every case, and in children should also be sent for cytogenetics. The biopsy should be done in a unit where there is experience of bone tumours and in particular where the pathologist is familiar with the very complex interpretation of bone tumour biopsies.

Management of patients with bone metastases

The most common tumours to metastasize to bone are breast, bronchus, thyroid, kidney and prostate, although any tumour can do this (even including sarcomas). The presence of bone metastases usually indicates the start of widespread tumour dissemination and treatment is mostly palliative, i.e. not curative. Metastases from prostate are frequently sclerotic whilst most other metastases are lytic and frequently lead to fracture. The most commonly affected bones are the spine, pelvis, ribs and femur.

The aim of orthopaedic management is to relieve symptoms, restore function and ensure that the patient has received appropriate supporting treatment from an oncologist. The prognosis for these patients is variable with a median survival of 3 months for patients with metastases from lung cancer but many years for patients with breast and renal metastases.

If a metastasis is detected prior to fracture, then the patient will usually receive oncological treatment depending on the primary (hormonal therapy and/or chemotherapy for some tumours, radiotherapy and bisphosphonates for most). Prophylactic fixation is indicated for persistent pain, particularly in a weight-bearing bone accompanied by destruction of the cortex.

If the bone has already fractured or if prophylactic fixation is used, it is essential to ensure that the fixation method used is sufficient to allow immediate restoration of function and should outlive the patient. More than half of pathological fractures will not heal and so whatever fixation is used, this must be taken into account. The use of joint replacements or custom prostheses is indicated for replacement of large areas of destroyed bone, particularly in patients with a reasonably good prognosis (solitary renal metastases and some breast metastases). If internal fixation devices are used, then intramedullary nails combined with the use of bone cement are preferred to plate and screw devices in most instances.

Patients with spinal metastases require careful assessment. If there is progressive pain, spinal collapse or neurological compromise, then spinal decompression and stabilization should be considered, especially in patients with a reasonable prognosis.

Patients should always be referred back to their oncologist for further management, which will usually include radiotherapy to the site of the metastasis to prevent recurrence.

Hamartomata

These are lesions of bone which are developmental but which often heal with time.

Fibrous cortical defect

Usually identified on an X-ray taken following trauma, these are usually asymptomatic defects in the cortex of bone which heal with skeletal maturity. They have typical radiological appearances and rarely need investigating. If the lesion is large or symptomatic, there is a small risk of fracture.

Fibrous dysplasia

This is a developmental abnormality of bone where the bone does not form properly and is weaker than normal. Stress fractures are common and in severe cases the bones can be bowed and deformed (e.g. the shepherd's crook deformity of the upper femur). X-rays typically show a ground-glass appearance

(see Fig. 9.1, p. 67). Treatment is conservative but, if a patient has persistent symptoms, then prophylactic stabilization may be helpful, often accompanied by curettage of the bone. Bisphosphonates may have a role in reducing symptoms for patients with polyostotic fibrous dysplasia.

Simple bone cysts

These typically arise in long bones in the skeletally immature patient and X-rays reveal a well-defined cyst in the bone. Spontaneous resolution by late adolescence is the rule. There is no guaranteed successful method of treatment, although there are claims for success by injection therapy with steroids or bone marrow, and others recommend curettage or bone grafting. In most cases avoidance of contact sports until the cyst heals is sufficient.

Benign bone tumours

Osteochondromas (exostoses)

These are the most common benign bone tumour. Most are solitary and are small bony outgrowths from the shaft of a long bone with a small cartilage cap. Symptoms arise from pressure on adjacent structures (e.g. muscle). Solitary osteochondromas can be removed if symptomatic. In the condition of *hereditary multiple exostoses (HME)* the patients have multiple lesions and the condition is inherited in a dominant fashion from one parent. These patients have a lifetime risk of one of the osteochondromas turning malignant (chondrosarcoma) of about 5–15%. The risk of malignancy in a solitary osteochondroma is low (probably <1 in 1000).

Aneurysmal bone cysts

These can look very similar to simple bone cysts, but can also arise in axial bones. Although spontaneous resolution can occur, most will progress if left and so treatment is recommended. Radiologically they can be indistinguishable from an osteosarcoma and biopsy should always be

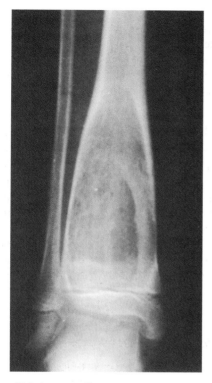

Figure 12.1 Aneurysmal bone cyst.

considered. Curettage alone leads to healing in over 90% of cases (Fig. 12.1).

Enchondromas

These are benign cartilage growths inside the bone. They are most common in the fingers but can also arise in the long bones where differentiation from a chondrosarcoma can be difficult. X-rays show popcorn calcification (Fig. 12.2). If an enchondroma is longer than 5 cm and is symptomatic, then potential malignancy should be considered. Asymptomatic enchondromas require no treatment, but small symptomatic ones are best treated with curettage.

Ollier's disease

The patient suffers from multiple enchondromas affecting many bones (see Fig. 9.2). The risk of

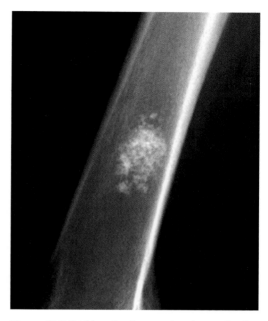

Figure 12.2 Radiograph of an enchondroma showing 'popcorn' calcification.

malignancy (chondrosarcoma) arising is about 10–15%. If the patient also has cutaneous angiomas then this is *Mafucci's syndrome* where the risk of malignancy is even higher.

Chondroblastoma

This is a benign cartilage tumour which typically arises in the epiphysis of the femur, tibia or humerus. Curettage is usually curative.

Chondromyxoid fibroma

This is a benign tumour typically arising eccentrically in the metaphysis of a long bone. Excision is usually curative.

Osteoid osteoma

This is a bone-forming tumour that typically arises in the cortex of a long bone. The mid-tibia is the most common site but any bone can be affected. The patient typically has a long history of pain,

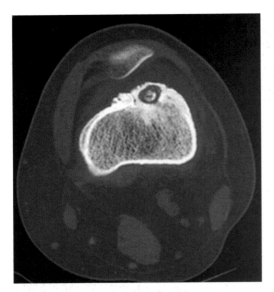

Figure 12.3 Osteoid osteoma showing central nidus.

especially at night, almost completely relieved by aspirin or other anti-inflammatory drug. X-rays show a central nidus with dense sclerosis around it (Fig. 12.3) and a bone scan is typically very hot. The cause is unknown and treatment consists of ablation of the nidus by radiofrequency or heat ablation under CT guidance.

Osteoblastomas

These are slightly larger versions of the same lesion and have a tendency to arise in the spine.

Giant cell tumours

These arise in the epiphysis after growth has finished and typically involve the knee region, with a lytic defect affecting either the femoral or tibial condyle extending right up to the joint line. They are called giant cell tumours because of the multinucleate giant cells which are in the tumour and which are stimulated to destroy bone. Biopsy is essential to exclude a malignant tumour. Treatment is by detailed curettage and can be supplemented with adjuncts such as phenol or cryotherapy followed by either bone grafting or cementation.

There is a 10–20% risk of local recurrence and a 1% risk of metastases developing, although these tend to behave very indolently. In some sites, excision and reconstruction may be appropriate and in others, such as the spine or pelvis, embolization, surgery and radiotherapy may be needed.

Primary malignant bone tumours

Osteosarcoma

This is a malignant neoplasm arising from bone cells which are undifferentiated and capable of forming bone, cartilage and collagenous tissue. It is the most commonly occurring primary tumour of bone, with an incidence of 3 per million population. It usually occurs under the age of 30, in boys more than in girls, and in cylindrical bones. The commonest bone affected is the femur (50%). The upper tibia and the upper end of the humerus are also common sites. It almost always affects the metaphysis. In older patients, typically over 50, it tends to occur in flat bones as well as long bones, and is then usually associated with Paget's disease or can be induced by previous radiotherapy.

Radiological features

The typical feature is a destructive lesion in the metaphysis—usually translucent and often with reactive periosteal new bone or rays of ossification within the expanding tumour ('sunburst effect') (Fig. 12.4). A soft-tissue mass may be apparent. Areas of calcification may occur, but are less evident than in chondrosarcoma.

Investigations

Staging is essential to assess both the local and distant extent of disease. As metastases tend to be blood borne, lung metastases are the greatest risk. All patients should have a CT chest and a bone scan to rule out metastatic disease.

Histologically, these tumours are pleomorphic with obvious malignant cells showing mitoses, but often with areas of bone, cartilage and fibrous tissue, which may confuse the diagnosis. The tumour is usually highly vascular, but there may be extensive necrosis. This variation in histological

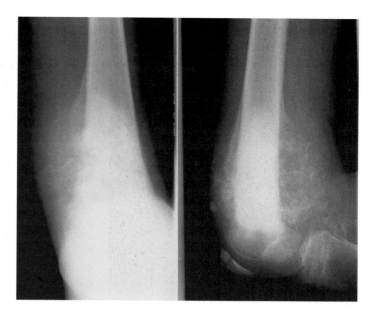

Figure 12.4 Osteosarcoma showing 'sunburst effect'.

pattern makes accurate diagnosis difficult and considerable experience is required in interpreting the sections.

Treatment

Treatment now almost always commences with chemotherapy. This has the advantage of immediately treating the micro-metastases which are almost certainly present by the time of diagnosis (but rarely detectable even with CT scanning of the lungs). Another advantage is that the primary tumour will often show some shrinkage. After 6–9 weeks, surgery is carried out. Limb salvage can often be achieved, i.e. resecting the tumour-bearing bone and surrounding soft tissues, the limb being reconstructed with a custom-built prosthesis and artificial joint if necessary. Survival appears to be no worse than after amputation and the procedure offers better palliation for those patients who already have pulmonary metastases. If the tumour is too extensive at the time of diagnosis and there is a poor response to chemotherapy, amputation may still be necessary. For patients with metastases at diagnosis, the prognosis is poor, but for those without detectable metastases, there is now a cure rate of 60%. Size of tumour and response to chemotherapy are the most important prognostic factors.

Osteosarcoma arising in Paget's disease is one of the most malignant tumours known and survival for 2 years is very unusual with any form of therapy. Patients with osteosarcoma arising after previous radiotherapy should be treated as a new primary osteosarcoma, although they may not be able to receive full doses of chemotherapy and surgery is usually more difficult.

Parosteal osteosarcoma is a low-grade osteosarcoma presenting with a dense calcified mass behind the knee. Complete surgical excision is required but chemotherapy is not needed in most cases.

Periosteal osteosarcoma is a conventional osteosarcoma arising under the periosteum. The tumours usually present early and treatment is surgical; the role of chemotherapy remains unclear.

Chondrosarcoma

This is a tumour which arises from chondroblasts and can only produce chondroid and collagen, not bone. It is rather more common in males. It typically affects the bones of the trunk and the proximal ends of long bones. It is unusual under the age of 30. Two types are seen—one arising within the bone (central) and the other on the

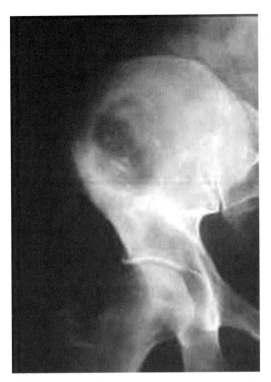

Figure 12.5 Chondrosarcoma.

surface (peripheral), sometimes in an osteochondroma. Benign chondromata in the digits rarely become malignant. The tumour may cause pain and a slowly increasing swelling, often over many years. Radiologically, it is represented by a translucent area, which may expand the bone (Fig. 12.5), and is often criss-crossed by spicules of calcification.

Complete surgical excision of the tumour is essential for cure as these tumours do not respond to surgery or chemotherapy. If the tumour is entered during excision, recurrence is more likely. Prognosis is related to the grade of the tumour (low grade doing best) and the ability to completely surgically remove it. *Dedifferentiated chondrosarcomas* arise when a conventional chondrosarcoma has an area of high-grade sarcoma adjacent to it. Surgical excision is essential but the prognosis is poor and there is no evidence of the effectiveness of chemotherapy.

Ewing's sarcoma

This is a malignant tumour arising in bone marrow, typically in patients under the age of 30. About two-thirds of the tumours occur in cylindrical bones, but the older the patient the more likely it is that the tumour arises in a flat bone because it develops from red marrow. It is not confined to the ends of long bones—a useful diagnostic point. There are about 80 cases per year in the UK and the cause is unknown.

Radiological features
The most striking feature is bone destruction and often a soft-tissue swelling. There may be some periosteal bone formation (Codman's triangle). Occasionally, there are onion-skin layers of new bone formation around the lesion. At diagnosis, 25% of patients will have metastases, either in the lung, other bones or bone marrow.

Diagnosis
Biopsy is essential. Occasionally, the centre of the tumour may be necrotic and liquefied, resembling pus. The tumour consists of round cells of uniform appearance—usually with areas of degeneration. The tumours have a characteristic t11:22 translocation on cytogenetic testing.

Treatment
Chemotherapy usually produces a dramatic response with necrosis of the tumour and resolution of symptoms. In most cases surgical resection of the residual primary site is recommended followed by radiotherapy unless there has been complete necrosis from the neoadjuvant chemotherapy. Survival rates approach 75% with poor prognostic factors being metastases at diagnosis, large tumours, poor response to chemotherapy and older patients.

Table 12.1 summarizes the features of these three most common malignant primary bone tumours.

Spindle cell sarcomas of bone

These are primary bone tumours which do not fit into one of the above categories. Although given a

Table 12.1 Features of malignant primary bone tumours.

	Age	Diagnosis	Radiology	Treatment	Prognosis
Osteosarcoma	<30	Femur in 50%, always metaphyseal, upper tibia and humerus common	Destructive with periosteal new bone	Chemotherapy then radical excision and replacement or amputation	60% survival if no metastases
Chondrosarcoma	>30	Bones of trunk and proximal ends of long bones	Translucent, spicules of bone	Surgical excision	Variable
Ewing's tumour	<30	Cylindrical bones. Biopsy, looks like pus	Periosteal reaction Onion-skin formation	Chemotherapy, then surgery and radiotherapy	75% survival

variety of histological names (e.g. fibrosarcoma, leiomyosarcoma, etc), they all behave in a similar manner to osteosarcoma, and should be treated the same way with chemotherapy and surgery.

Haematological malignancies

Non-Hodgkin's lymphoma

This is a destructive bone tumour of adults, rather like Ewing's sarcoma, both radiologically and histologically, but with a better prognosis. Chemotherapy has again improved the survival rate and radiotherapy will usually control the bone involved.

Plasmacytoma and myeloma

A plasmacytoma is a solitary form of myeloma, both being tumours of plasma cells. Treatment for plasmacytoma is usually with radiotherapy, but if the patient develops systemic disease (myeloma), chemotherapy may be indicated. In myeloma the patients have elevated serum immunoglobulins and may have Bence Jones protein in the urine. The bone lesions usually respond well to radiotherapy, but in some cases stabilization or occasionally replacement of a very damaged bone is required.

Soft-tissue sarcomas

These can arise from any tissue within the body. Their incidence is approximately 60 per million per year (3000 per year in the UK) of which half occur in the musculoskeletal system. There are no

Box 12.3 Features suggesting malignancy.

- Lump >5 cm
- Increasing in size
- Recently painful
- Deep to fascia
- Recurrence after previous excision

specific clinical features suggesting malignancy in any lump, but Box 12.3 lists features which are highly suggestive.

Any lump exhibiting one or more of these features should be investigated to rule out malignancy—usually by cross-sectional imaging (MRI) and biopsy (ideally needle biopsy). There are a wide range of histological types of soft-tissue sarcoma, the most common being liposarcoma, leiomyosarcoma, synovial sarcoma and rhabdomyosarcoma. Many have no particular distinguishing feature and are known as 'spindle cell sarcomas'.

The management of soft-tissue sarcomas is by surgical excision with a wide margin around the tumour, usually followed by radiotherapy. 'Shell-out' procedures are unacceptable and result, almost inevitably, in local recurrence. Amputation may sometimes be necessary for large tumours. Despite these measures, metastases (usually in the lungs) occur in 50% of patients and in these cases the outlook is bleak. Chemotherapy has little role at the present time for most soft-tissue sarcomas. The prognosis is related to the histological grade and the size of the tumour, as well as the age of the patient.

Chapter 13

Infections

Soft-tissue infections

These can generally be regarded as either community acquired or hospital acquired (nosocomial), such as infected surgical wounds, cannula sites, etc. The distinction is important when considering likely causative organisms and choosing empiric antibiotic regimes (e.g. meticillin-resistant *Staphylococcus aureus* may be more prominent in hospital). Skin and soft-tissue infections can range in magnitude from mild to severe and life-threatening, and range in depth from superficial infections, such as impetigo and erysipelas, to infection of the deeper structures, such as cellulitis and fasciitis.

Cellulitis

This is a spreading infection of the soft tissues, often caused by a β-haemolytic streptococci, most notably the Group A streptococcus (*Streptococcus pyogenes*) and less commonly by other organisms, including *Staph. aureus*, or sometimes polymicrobial in nature. The infected area is painful, hot and oedematous, usually with lymphangitis. There is usually no localization of the infection or pus for-

mation and the initial source of infection is often not apparent (insect bites, athlete's foot or trauma, such as ill-fitting shoes all serve as potential sources). The patient may be pyrexial, which is associated with the toxaemia from the streptococcal (sometimes staphylococcal) toxins.

Treatment

Antibiotic therapy is usually adequate, but cases of necrotizing fasciitis may present along similar lines, and in these cases, surgery is essential and life-saving (an early cardinal sign of necrotizing fasciitis is pain, more than would often be expected from the visible extent of the infection).

Penicillin remains the most appropriate antibiotic for streptococcal infection. Oral penicillins often achieve poor tissue levels and amoxicillin is preferable, with oral penicillin reserved for treatment of pharyngitis/tonsillitis, provided the patient is not allergic to it. In cases of allergy, then local prescribing guidelines or a clinical microbiologist should be consulted. Healing in cases of cellulitis is usually complete.

Abscess

Many infections, particularly of wounds and penetrating injuries, with or without a foreign body, eventually become localized to form an abscess. Drainage (often with antibiotic cover) is usually curative. The possibility of a fungal or parasitic

Lecture Notes: Orthopaedics and Fractures, 4e.
By T Duckworth and CM Blundell. Published 2010 by Blackwell Publishing.

infection should be remembered, particularly with tropical soft-tissue abscesses. A swinging pyrexia is classically regarded as indicating a collection of pus. Natural or surgical drainage is usually necessary if an abscess has formed. A foreign body, such as a fragment of soil, clothing or metallic implant, may cause a persistent sinus until it is removed.

Wound infections

Infection of wounds is common, but less likely to occur if adequate wound toilet has been performed with removal of dead or devitalized tissues and foreign material. Post-operative wound infections are often related to tissue damage or to haematoma formation. Infection should be suspected if the patient is pyrexial and the wound is tense, inflamed and oedematous. In hospitalized patients, consider infection of line/cannula sites also, in which case line removal and cultures (blood, line tip and possibly swab of the site) are required, as well as appropriate empiric antibiotics, dictated by local antibiotic policy.

Clostridial infections

A variety of organisms belonging to the Clostridium genus can cause soft-tissue infections. The often problematic *C. difficile*, which whilst not being associated with skin and soft-tissue infections, can frequently be seen as a cause of diarrhoea (and occasionally colitis). *C. difficile* is usually associated with the use of antibiotics (skin and soft-tissue infections are amongst the commonest reasons for the prescribing of antibiotics). Although commoner in the hospital setting, this can also be encountered in the community, including long-term care facilities.

Tetanus

This is a serious form of wound infection caused by spores of the *C. tetani* bacillus which have been implanted in the wound, often by contamination with soil. The organism is anaerobic and dead tissue is a favourable environment for its growth. The entry wound may sometimes be no more than a puncture. This infection can also be seen in the

tropics where it can be associated with super-infection of relatively minor trauma wounds on the feet and legs, or secondary infection of tropical ulcers.

The incubation period is from 2 days to 3 weeks. A powerful neurotoxin is produced, causing tonic and clonic muscle contractions. These spasms may develop first at the site of infection and quickly and characteristically involve the facial and jaw muscles, producing 'lockjaw' and 'risus sardonicus'. There is then gradual spread of muscle involvement and eventually respiratory arrest. The early symptoms may be mild, usually stiffness of the jaw, neck and back muscles. Usually the shorter the incubation time, the worse the prognosis.

Active immunization with toxoid is now usually provided from school age. Following any penetrating injury occurring more than 5 years after active immunization, a booster dose is given. If the interval is more than 10 years, a new course is started and 250 units of human tetanus immunoglobulin are also given. Adequate wound toilet with excision of dead tissue is an important preventive measure. Treatment of the established case requires the anaesthetic facilities of an intensive care unit.

Gas gangrene

An uncommon condition caused by the anaerobic bacillus *C. perfringens* and occasionally by other clostridia. It usually occurs in wounds contaminated by soil and manure, especially if necrotic tissue is present. It causes gas to form in the tissues with a red discoloration of the skin, a foul smelling discharge, and spreading gangrene. The toxin is potentially lethal, but anti-serum and early wide excision of dead muscle or amputation may be life-saving. Hyperbaric oxygen has been advocated but its value remains uncertain.

Wound botulism

This has been seen in recent years in association with intravenous drug usage, where spore-contaminated batches of heroin have been injected directly into tissues (so called 'skin popping'). The acidic nature of the injected drug creates local tissue necrosis where the spores of the *C. botulinum* bacillus can germinate and eventually produce their neurotoxin. The toxin itself, whilst being of similar nature to the tetanus toxin, causes the opposite effect and primarily manifests as weakness from the blockade of the peripheral neuromuscular junction and autonomic synapses. The classical presentation is that of bilateral cranial neuropathies associated with symmetrical descending weakness. The Centers for Disease Control and Prevention (CDC) list the cardinal features as: absence of fever usually, symmetrical neurological manifestations, patient remains responsive, heart rate normal or slow and, except for blurred vision, no sensory deficit.

Good supportive care (intensive care and intubation), soft-tissue debridement, appropriate antibiotics (including metronidazole) and administration of anti-toxin are the cornerstones of treatment.

Bone and joint infections

Acute osteomyelitis

This is a common condition and is usually caused by *Staph. pyogenes*, but occasionally by other organisms, e.g. streptococcus, pneumococcus, salmonella and *Escherichia coli*.

It occurs mainly in children. Poor living conditions predispose to it, and there may be an obvious primary focus of infection, such as a boil, sore throat, etc.

There is often a history of preceding injury and some patients may develop infection in a subperiosteal haematoma.

Pathology

The infection usually starts in the vascular metaphysis of a long bone or in the centre of a short bone. Common sites are the lower end of the femur and upper end of the tibia, either end of the humerus, radius and ulna, and the vertebral bodies. Because of the confined space and tension, tissue necrosis occurs readily and an abscess may form within the bone. The pus usually breaks out under the periosteum, stripping it and eventually penetrating to a point on the surface (Fig. 13.1).

Large areas of bone may become necrotic, making penetration by antibiotics difficult and forming 'sequestra' or hidden areas of dead and infected bone. These may act as foreign bodies,

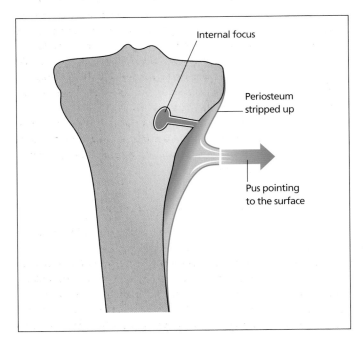

Internal focus

Periosteum stripped up

Pus pointing to the surface

Figure 13.1 Acute osteomyelitis.

> **Box 13.1** Clinical features of acute osteomyelitis.
>
> - Fever—acute onset with malaise
> - Pain—localized to metaphysis classically
> - Swelling—often associated with joint stiffness
> - Tenderness—localized
> - Oedema and pus (late sign)—pus may break through the periosteum, causing a fluctuant mass

maintaining the sepsis in chronic form. If the centre of the shaft becomes infected, the nutrient artery may thrombose, leading to sequestration of the whole shaft. In this case, if the patient survives, the sequestrated shaft may become surrounded by a shell of new bone, with holes through which pus may continue to find its way to the surface, forming persistent sinuses. This shell is called an involucrum. With improved management this complication is now rarely seen.

Clinical features

These are listed in Box 13.1.

Swelling of nearby joints is usually due to a 'sympathetic' effusion. Occasionally, especially if the metaphysis is intracapsular, the joint itself may become infected.

The condition can also be seen in neonates and is difficult to diagnose, often remaining almost silent. The baby usually fails to thrive and cries when the limb is moved.

Management

Urgent treatment is required if the condition is suspected and includes:

1 Blood culture

2 Broad-spectrum antibiotics (the exact combination will depend upon local policy). Initially these are often given parenterally.

The antibiotics usually control the septicaemia and fever quite quickly.

1 If given early enough, the antibiotics may control the infection and complete healing may then take place with re-absorption of small sequestra.

2 Pus formation may already have occurred by the time treatment has started. In this case, the temperature usually starts to swing after first settling

on antibiotic treatment. The pain and swelling persist. Localized oedema of the skin is a useful sign of pus formation. Fluctuation is often difficult to detect.

3 If pus is suspected, surgical drainage is necessary. Pus may break through the periosteum or this may need to be incised.

4 Following drainage, antibiotics can be continued or changed according to the culture result (broad-spectrum agents can be switched to a more narrow-spectrum agent). If the condition then settles, a total of 6 weeks' antibiotic therapy is usually recommended. The erythrocyte sedimentation rate (ESR) is a guide to recovery during this period. The majority of children are cured by this regime and recurrence is unusual.

Osteomyelitis of the spine

This may be difficult to diagnose and is often less acute than with other sites. Fevers with bone pain and muscle spasm are usual. Walking may be difficult and painful. The disease typically affects the vertebral bodies, but may affect the posterior elements.

Diagnosis may need blood culture and aspiration or drainage of pus from a paravertebral abscess. Cord symptoms are rare but serious. Acute osteomyelitis of the spine is usually secondary to bacteraemic spread; common sources include skin and soft-tissue infections, cannula/line-associated infections, urinary tract infection, endocarditis and respiratory tract infection.

Treatment relies on prolonged antibiotics (preferably against an identified pathogen from biopsy or blood culture) and surgical drainage where necessary.

Acute suppurative arthritis

This is a serious and damaging condition, which arises (Box 13.2):

1 From progression of osteomyelitis, usually in joints where the metaphysis is intracapsular—especially the hip and upper end of the radius. Occasionally, in older children spread occurs through the epiphyseal plate into the epiphysis

> **Box 13.2** Pathogenesis of acute suppurative arthritis.
>
> - Spread of osteomyelitis (hip and elbow)
> - Haematogenous (infants especially)
> - Inflammatory arthritides
> - Penetrating 'injuries' (including joint injections)

and then into the joint itself. Osteomyelitis of the acetabulum may be difficult to distinguish from septic arthritis

2 From haematogenous spread, particularly in infants, where multiple joint infections may occur and be relatively silent

3 In rheumatoid joints, especially in patients on steroids. The infection may arise by haematogenous spread or by direct implantation from an intra-articular injection, particularly if a steroid has been injected

4 Following penetrating injuries.

The infection is usually staphylococcal but may be by other organisms. The synovium becomes inflamed and thickened; fluid is increased and quickly becomes purulent. Muscle spasm and softening of ligaments and capsule may allow dislocation (especially of the hip in an infant—Smith's arthritis). Pus eventually ruptures through the capsule and points, but by then the articular cartilage is usually severely damaged. In the hip the increased pressure may cause ischaemic necrosis of the femoral head.

The patient is usually ill with high fever and rigors due to septicaemia. The joint is acutely painful and swollen, and is hot and very tender. There is almost always extreme muscle spasm, often allowing no movement of the joint or the limb. The differential diagnosis is from osteomyelitis with a sympathetic effusion, rheumatic fever, rheumatoid arthritis or Still's disease (usually multiple joints), Reiter's syndrome and gout.

Radiology

There may be no X-ray changes in the early stages. Later, sub-periosteal new bone may become visible with generalized periarticular porosis. Pathological subluxation or dislocation may occur and this may

be difficult to diagnose in the infant whose epiphyses are not yet ossified.

Management

To establish a diagnosis, the joint should be aspirated on suspicion. The organisms may be identified by culture of blood and the joint aspirate (a negative Gram film does not exclude infection and should not necessarily be relied upon to guide antibiotic choice). The choice of antibiotic will depend upon local prescribing policy and is usually continued for 6 weeks.

The infected joint is usually subject to a surgical washout, depending upon the degree and severity of infection, and an orthopaedic opinion regarding this should be sought early.

Septic arthritis arising secondary to penetrating injuries and open wounds is usually less destructive, and although drainage may be required, a mobile joint may often be preserved.

Chronic infection

Chronic paronychia

This is a persistent nailfold infection usually caused by a fungus or by repeated irritation, e.g. with detergents. It does not suppurate and usually responds to anti-fungal agents given locally or systemically. Herpes simplex virus (HSV) is the causative organism for the herpetic whitlow, which is usually soft tissue in nature and is often caused from auto-inoculation (from a facial HSV infection/re-activation or cold sore).

Chronic infections of the nails

These are often fungal and result in discoloration and deformities of the nail. They can often be eradicated by oral anti-fungal agents.

Chronic pyogenic osteomyelitis

This is an uncommon, localized bone infection arising from one of the following situations:

1 After trauma to bone, e.g. open fracture or penetrating injury. Bullet wounds with much contamination are particularly liable to result in pyogenic osteomyelitis

2 By haematogenous spread, the source of which may remain unknown. The infection may take the form of a cavity in the bone with surrounding sclerosis, giving rise to intermittent attacks of pain—Brodie's abscess. It may contain pus but organisms are not always cultivated (especially if there has been prior antibiotic exposure)

3 As a result of inadequately treated acute osteomyelitis. In the typical case the infection is perpetuated by necrosis of bone, often resulting in sequestra ranging in size from a few millimetres to almost the whole shaft. The living bone becomes thickened and honeycombed and may surround the sequestrum completely, preventing its discharge (involucrum)

4 As a complication of surgery, particularly when foreign material is implanted. The infection usually results in failure of the implant.

Clinical course

The disease is characterized by 'flares' of infection with pain and swelling, and often pus formation, alternating with periods of quiescence, sometimes lasting several years. Occasionally, particularly following penetrating injuries, open fractures and replacement arthroplasty, a sinus may form and discharge continuously. Often when the discharge stops the condition becomes acute until the resulting abscess is drained.

Investigations

X-rays demonstrate the abnormal bone texture with thickening and diffuse cavity formation (Fig. 13.2). A sequestrum usually shows up as a localized mass of bone, denser than its surroundings. Culture of the pus from a persistent sinus usually yields mixed organisms from secondary infection. The ESR is raised and the white cell count shows a moderate leucocytosis.

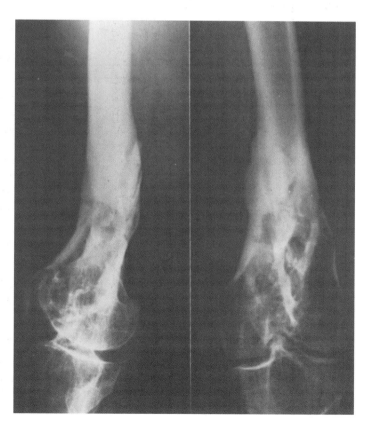

Figure 13.2 Chronic osteomyelitis following an open fracture.

Treatment

This is difficult and consists of the following.

1 Treating acute episodes with the appropriate antibiotic, which is usually known from previous culture. Surgical drainage may be necessary.

2 Attempts at eradication. This is often impossible, but long-term antibiotics combined with excision of sequestra and opening up of poorly draining cavities may be successful. For the extensively involved bone, the procedure of 'guttering', which involves opening the medullary cavity widely and allowing the wound to granulate and heal from the bottom, used to be popular. Newer methods involve opening the bone widely, scraping out cavities and closing the defect with muscle on a vascular pedicle or a split-skin or pedicle-skin graft. There is interest in removing the infected segment completely and closing the gap by performing an osteotomy some distance away and transporting the healthy bone to fill the gap using an Ilizarov frame and bone lengthening techniques. A technique whereby the medullary canal is continuously lavaged with a system of tubing with antibiotics in the wash for several weeks (Lautenbach procedure) has been described but is the remit of specialist bone infection units.

Chronic osteomyelitis occurring as a complication of replacement arthroplasty presents formidable problems and is becoming increasingly common.

3 Amputation may occasionally be required.

Tuberculosis of bones and joints

Two strains of tubercle bacillus are responsible, human and bovine. Bone and joint tuberculosis usually occurs in the later stages of the generalized disease. The initial infection is either via the respiratory tract or the intestine, and the bacilli reach the spine or limbs by blood spread.

Incidence

Worldwide resurgence of tuberculosis over the last few decades now makes TB one of the leading causes of death worldwide. The highest incidence of TB is in immigrants from parts of the world where TB is endemic (and HIV also as the two

infections have gone hand in hand), most especially sub-Saharan Africa, parts of the Far East and the Indian sub-continent. Drug-resistant TB is an increasing global problem.

Pathology

The prominent features are:

1 Destruction of bone and articular cartilage by tuberculous granulation tissue with areas of healing by fibrosis

2 Thickening of synovial membrane which becomes studded with tubercles and extends as a pannus under the edges of the articular cartilage, destroying it

3 Abscess formation, especially in spinal tuberculosis. The pus tracks along tissue planes, particularly within the psoas sheath in association with spinal infections and may point some distance from the original site, e.g. in the groin. Spread can occur through cartilaginous epiphyses and endplates and across the intervertebral discs

4 Fibrosis occurs in the healing phase. The joint may remain mobile or may develop a fibrous or bony ankylosis (Fig. 13.3).

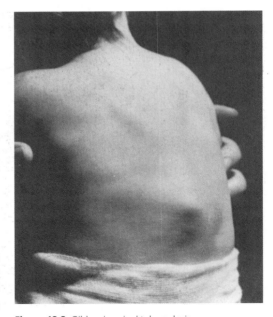

Figure 13.3 Gibbus in spinal tuberculosis.

Clinical features

Infection of bone alone is unusual, occasionally occurring in metacarpals, phalanges, ribs or greater trochanter. Usually, the infection involves both bone and joints:

1 Starting in the metaphysis as in acute osteomyelitis and spreading to the joint, especially when the metaphysis is intracapsular; or
2 Starting in the synovial membrane.

In both cases the whole joint and bone ends are quickly affected.

X-ray appearances

1 Osteoporotic changes around the joint may be the first sign.
2 Erosion of the joint surfaces with decreased joint space.
3 Destruction of bone (and intervertebral discs).
4 Soft-tissue shadows representing abscesses, e.g. the 'bird's nest' shadow of a paravertebral abscess which is almost always present in spinal tuberculosis (Fig. 13.4).

Investigations

1 The ESR is usually raised and is an index of progress.

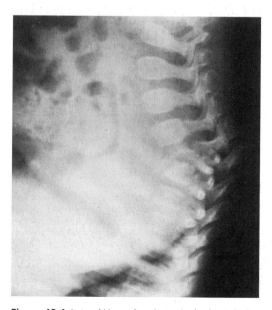

Figure 13.4 Lateral X-ray showing spinal tuberculosis.

2 Moderate lymphocytosis is usual.
3 The tuberculin (Mantoux or Heaf) test may be positive (except in early cases who rarely have bone and joint TB). Very occasionally, a patient with widespread 'miliary' tuberculosis may be tuberculin negative and the same can be true in those individuals with HIV infection.
4 Biopsy of lymph glands may show typical tuberculosis, but biopsy of bone or synovium is usually more reliable, allowing histological examination and TB culture (most UK laboratories now employ a liquid medium-based rapid culture system which usually can yield positive results within 2 weeks).
5 Bacilli may be cultured from sputum (including induced or obtained via bronchoscopy).

Treatment

Infection is always generalized and drug therapy is the key element of treatment. It can usually be started before waiting for final confirmation of the diagnosis. It must be emphasized, however, that because of the risks of encouraging the emergence of drug-resistant strains, it is absolutely essential that drug therapy be controlled by careful sensitivity testing of the organisms and hence tissue (and usually sputum) for culture is mandatory.

The currently recommended regime uses rifampicin, isoniazid, pyrazinamide and often, initially at least, ethambutol. The usual regime is to start with a three- or four-drug combination and subsequently reduce this to two on the basis of the sensitivities. Anti-tubercle drugs should never be used as a monotherapy due to the high rate of resistance associated with this. A 6-month course is usual for pulmonary TB, but longer periods are required for extra-pulmonary disease. Expert assistance from a TB specialist should be sought before embarking on TB treatment.

Sinuses

A sinus is a blind track communicating with an epithelial surface such as the skin or an internal organ. The track itself may be lined with epithelium. Chronic infection may play a part in the persistence of a sinus, sometimes secondary to the underlying pathology. A sinus may form for several reasons.

1 Congenital. These usually represent the persistence of an embryological structure, e.g. a branchial or thyroglossal sinus.

2 Foreign body. This may be material which is foreign to the body, or dead tissue which may behave as a foreign body, particularly if infected. A bony sequestrum is an example of this. Healing will rarely occur once infection is established, until the foreign material is removed. This is particularly a problem with infected prostheses.

3 Chronic infection. Such chronic conditions as tuberculosis, fungal infections, etc may produce a chronic sinus after the abscess has discharged or been drained.

4 Neoplasia. Rarely, a sinus may communicate with a neoplastic mass. A long-established chronic sinus may itself develop secondary neoplastic changes.

Antibiotic regimes

Given the variations which exist not only in local, regional and sometimes national antibiotic prescribing policies, as well as variations in rates of antibiotic resistance, specific antibiotic regimes have not generally been recommended, as they will no doubt be subject to change. Consultation of local policy or discussion with the local microbiologist is therefore recommended instead.

Chapter 14

Metabolic diseases of bone

In addition to its supporting function, bone acts as an important organ in controlling the metabolism of calcium and phosphate in the body.

Calcium metabolism

The skeleton contains 98% of the body's calcium. The daily turnover of calcium is represented diagrammatically in Figure 14.1. Calcium is interchanged between the body pool, the gut, kidneys and bone, and in normal circumstances the amount excreted balances the amount taken in by the diet. Many factors influence this system.

1 Parathyroid hormone. This is a polypeptide and its output is determined by the serum calcium level, increasing when the calcium level is low. It restores the calcium level to normal by increasing tubular re-absorption from the kidney and mobilizing calcium from the bones.

2 Calcitonin. This hormone is produced by the C-cells of the thyroid gland. Its precise role is disputed, but it inhibits bone resorption and is secreted in response to a raised serum calcium.

3 Vitamin D. Cholecalciferol is a fat-soluble vitamin contained in many fatty foods, notably milk and fish-liver oils, and it is also synthesized in the skin by the action of sunlight. It is converted to 25-hydroxycholecalciferol in the liver by the addition of an OH radical and is further converted in the kidney to 1,25-dihydroxycholecalciferol (1,25-DHCC). Other conversions are also possible in the kidney, although 1,25-DHCC appears to be the main metabolically active one. The active vitamin affects:

- Gut—increases calcium absorption
- Bone—indirectly affects both bone deposition and resorption
- Muscle—muscle weakness occurs in vitamin D deficiency.

Increased levels of 1,25-DHCC tend to increase both calcium and phosphate levels in the serum. Because the active metabolites are produced in the kidney, renal failure may produce the effects of vitamin D deficiency, and this can only be overcome by giving large doses of cholecalciferol or, alternatively, giving the more active metabolites.

In vitamin D deficiency, the parathyroids are stimulated to restore the calcium levels—secondary hyperparathyroidism.

These hormonal effects are summarized in Table 14.1.

These and many other factors influence bone formation and deposition. Imbalance between them causes either increased or decreased bone mass. The understanding of these bone changes has been confused by the use of imprecise terms.

Lecture Notes: Orthopaedics and Fractures, 4e.
By T Duckworth and CM Blundell. Published 2010 by Blackwell Publishing.

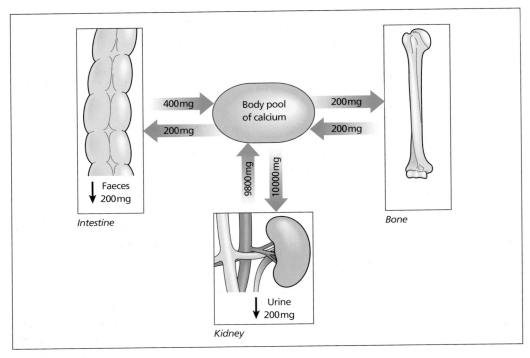

Figure 14.1 Calcium pool.

Table 14.1 Hormonal influences on serum calcium.

Hormone	Mechanism	Controlled by	Effect
Parathyroid hormone	Mobilizes Ca^{2+} from bone Increases renal re-absorption of Ca^{2+}	Serum calcium	↑Serum calcium
Calcitonin	Inhibits bone resorption Reduces renal re-absorption of Ca^{2+} Decreases gut absorption of Ca^{2+}	Serum calcium	↓Serum calcium
Vitamin D	Increases gut Ca^{2+} absorption Changes bone turnover	Diet Sunlight Renal function	↑Serum calcium

The classification below is that suggested by Aegeter and Kirkpatrick.

Bone loss

Bone loss (with decreased radiological density and usually thinning of the cortex) can be due to:
1 Decrease in osteoid formation (osteopenia)
2 Decrease in mineralization of osteoid (osteomalacia) or

3 Increase in removal of bone by osteoclasts (osteolysis).

Osteopenia

Dietary causes

Deficient intake of vitamins or essential proteins may occur in the malabsorption syndromes, and rarely from a true dietary deficiency, e.g. scurvy.

Scurvy/vitamin C deficiency

This has become rare and only occurs in the fully developed form in children between the ages of 6 months and 1 year, although old people may have a sub-clinical deficiency. Vitamin C is necessary for collagen synthesis and osteoid deposition, especially at the growing ends of bones.

Pathological features

In the long bones the zone of provisional calcification occurs as usual and appears on X-ray as a dense band at the epiphysis with an adjacent lucent band representing deficient osteoid formation. The epiphysis is ringed with a zone of calcification. Capillaries are abnormally fragile, causing soft-tissue haemorrhages, often under the periosteum at the ends of long bones and in the soft tissues. These particularly affect the gums and skin. Fractures and epiphyseal displacements are common, and unite with enormous amounts of callus. Wounds may be slow to heal.

Treatment

Ascorbic acid treatment is rapidly curative.

Endocrine causes

Cushing's syndrome or steroid therapy

Both of these cause a generalized osteopenia, often with crush fractures in vertebrae. Steroid therapy over a long period may also cause ischaemic necrosis of epiphyses, notably the femoral head. This is a problem in patients who have had organ transplants, or other conditions requiring long-term steroids for immunosuppression, such as inflammatory arthritis.

Hyperthyroidism

Detectable osteopenia occurs uncommonly.

Disuse atrophy

Bone formation is responsive to mechanical stress, and a period of immobilization in a plaster-cast or of enforced bed rest may lead to localized or generalized osteopenia.

> **Box 14.1** Causes of osteomalacia.
>
> - Lack of vitamin D or calcium (rickets)
> - Renal tubular acidosis
> - Parathyroid hormone insufficiency

Osteogenesis imperfecta

See Chapter 9.

Osteomalacia

This is a failure of bone mineralization which may lead to pain, weakness and fragility of the bone. Causes are given in Box 14.1.

Rickets

This is a childhood form of osteomalacia. Its effects are due to failure of bone mineral to ossify from lack of vitamin D. Dietary deficiency has now become rare except in economically deprived countries, particularly where there is also deficient exposure to sunlight.

In growing bones the failure of ossification leads to widening of the epiphyseal lines and generalized demineralization. The epiphyses are widened and have a 'cupped' appearance, usually best seen on an AP radiograph of the wrist.

Clinical features

Symptoms usually start about the age of 1. The child is small and fails to thrive, developing deformities such as bowing of the femora and tibiae, a large head and deformity of the chest with thickening of the costochondral junctions (ricketty rosary) and a transverse sulcus in the chest caused by the pull of the diaphragm (Harrison's sulcus) (Fig. 14.2).

Investigations

The serum calcium is usually normal, the phosphate is low and the alkaline phosphatase is raised.

Treatment

Ordinary doses of vitamin D are curative.

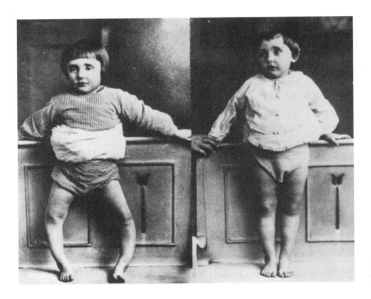

Figure 14.2 Rickets before and after treatment.

Renal rickets and vitamin D-resistant rickets

As described above, renal disease may interfere with vitamin D metabolism, diminishing the production of the more active derivatives. This may result in malabsorption and abnormal utilization of calcium and phosphate, with secondary parathyroid stimulation and consequent further demineralization. The effects are complex.

Certain types of renal tubular insufficiency may result in reduced re-absorption of phosphate, causing hypophosphataemia and secondary bone demineralization.

Both the above types of rickets are resistant to normal doses of vitamin D, but may respond to enormous doses or to the more active metabolites, such as 1,25-DHCC. Large and repeated doses of phosphate may be valuable in the second type.

The orthopaedic problems are the same as those of ordinary rickets, with similar bone deformities and also a tendency to fragmentation and slipping of the femoral head, resulting in coxa vara.

The deformities of all types of rickets may be corrected, if necessary, when the disease is under control. Prophylactic pinning of the slipping femoral neck may be useful in renal rickets, although the prognosis for life is poor.

Adult osteomalacia

The changes are mainly those of softening of the bones. The effects on the growing epiphyses do not apply in the adult so that deformities are not usually severe. The condition is probably more common than is usually thought, particularly in older people who may have dietary deficiency and do not receive sufficient sunlight.

In Britain, the condition is commonly found in Asian immigrants whose diet may be deficient and may also encourage calcium deficiency, e.g. phytic acid in the flour used to make chappatis combines with calcium to make it unabsorbable.

Clinical and radiological features

1 Generalized bone pain with occasional exacerbations usually in the spine due to crush fractures.

2 Anorexia, weight loss, muscle weakness, sometimes bony deformity.

3 X-rays show diffuse osteoporosis, pathological vertebral wedging and pseudo-fractures, which are translucent zones with surrounding sclerosis, usually running at right angles to the margin of the bone (Looser's zones). They are well seen in the vertebral border of the scapula and the ischio-pubic ramus.

Diagnosis

Serum calcium and phosphate may be lowered. Alkaline phosphatase is raised. Iliac crest bone biopsy is useful and shows the typical unmineralized osteoid 'seams' lying against normally calcified areas.

Treatment

Vitamin D in normal doses or, more effectively, a more active metabolite, is usually rapidly curative.

Osteolysis

Here, the loss of mineralized bone is due to osteoclastic resorption in excess of deposition. The most potent factor producing this is over-activity of parathyroid secretion.

Hyperparathyroidism

Three types are recognized:

1 Primary hyperparathyroidism, due either to generalized hyperplasia of the parathyroid or to an adenoma.

2 Secondary hyperparathyroidism, usually in response to renal disease or as a sequel to osteomalacia or malabsorption. The parathyroid hormone acts to restore serum calcium and phosphate levels by causing demineralization.

3 Tertiary hyperparathyroidism is the expression used to describe the situation where the constantly stimulated gland of secondary hyperparathyroidism develops an autonomous over-secretion so that even if the underlying cause is eliminated, the gland may still over-secrete.

In primary hyperparathyroidism the serum calcium in blood and urine is raised and phosphate lowered. In secondary hyperparathyroidism calcium may be normal or even low, and phosphate levels vary, depending on the renal pathology.

Primary hyperparathyroidism

This is characterized by generalized skeletal porosis and the development of cystic lesions filled with soft brown connective tissue. These usually occur in the long bones, but are not always present.

Because of these cysts, the disease is sometimes called osteitis fibrosa cystica.

Clinical features

These consist of generalized bone pains, indigestion, weakness and anorexia. Fractures and deformities complicate the condition. Renal calculi may occur and eventually renal failure.

Radiological features

There is generalized porosis and characteristic localized lesions, which are usually well circumscribed in long bones. These may be widespread or few in number (Fig. 14.3). A lateral radiograph of the skull may show a characteristic 'pepper pot' appearance which is virtually diagnostic.

Diagnosis

This rests on high serum calcium, low phosphate and raised alkaline phosphatase. Bone biopsy may be helpful.

Treatment

In the primary case, the parathyroid adenoma may be excised. Generalized hyperplasia, if it is primary, may require removal of two or more of the glands.

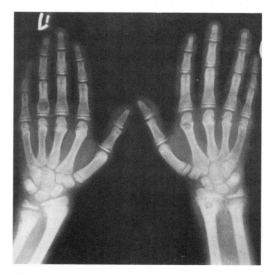

Figure 14.3 Osteitis fibrosa cystica.

Osteoporosis

As commonly used, this term is based on clinical and radiological findings rather than on pathology. It is most common in old age and particularly in post-menopausal women, although men are not immune. It is defined as a reduction in bone mineral density as a result of reduced mineral mass, as well as a change in the micro-architecture of the bone itself.

Its causes probably include dietary deficiency, lack of stress on bones, both of which cause osteopenia or osteomalacia, and hormonal changes which may act by influencing the effect of parathyroid hormone and therefore allowing osteolysis. In other words, all the mechanisms of reduction of mineralized bone mass may apply.

Clinical features

It usually affects women over 60 and to a lesser extent men of the same age. Occasionally, symptoms become marked at or soon after the menopause. The clinical features are bone pains, lassitude and acute back pain due to pathological vertebral fractures. The gradual development of a kyphosis and loss of height are the main features. Hip fractures in the aged are almost certainly related to osteoporosis.

Diagnosis

All patients should be screened biochemically and radiologically to attempt to exclude the specific disorders listed above.

In typical senile or post-menopausal osteoporosis the X-rays show generalized loss of density of bones and thinning of the cortices from within. The bones may have a 'ghostly' quality. Vertebrae may be wedged or the discs may protrude into the bodies ('ballooning' of the disc) (Fig. 14.4). Kyphosis is usual and stress fractures may occur.

It is now possible to assess the degree of osteoporosis by measuring bone density using a dual-energy X-ray absorptiometric device, known as the DEXA scanner, and this is used as a screening technique to detect patients at risk, particularly post-menopausal women.

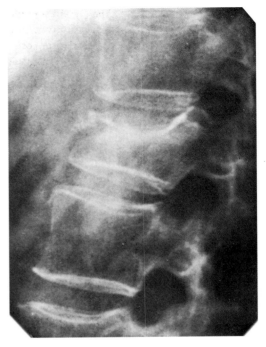

Figure 14.4 Osteoporotic spine with wedge fracture.

Histological features

The Haversian canals are widened and the trabeculae are thin and sparse. The bone which is present is usually adequately mineralized, but there may be occasional 'osteoid seams'.

Treatment

Treatment and prophylaxis are controversial. It is usual to give the patient an orthopaedic support for the spine, to encourage exercise and to give dietary supplements of calcium, vitamin D and proteins, although the effects of the latter are probably marginal. Oestrogen therapy, often called 'hormone replacement therapy' (HRT), is now accepted as a useful method of prophylaxis for peri- and post-menopausal women identified by screening as being particularly at risk. Compliance is often poor, particularly if a formulation which causes post-menopausal bleeding is used, and there have been fears of precipitating breast and uterine cancer.

Androgen therapy has also been tried with little proven benefit. High fluoride levels in drinking water are associated with a lower incidence of osteoporosis so fluoride therapy has been advocated, but it has been shown to be associated with a high incidence of hip fracture. Newer forms of treatment have included calcitonin and bisphosphonates, which have been shown to reduce the risks of osteoporotic fractures. Many forms of treatment can be shown to influence the biochemistry of osteoporotic patients, but it is difficult to prove that they influence the condition of the bones or that they alleviate symptoms.

Chapter 15

Examination of the musculoskeletal system

History taking

The art of taking a good history lies in eliciting as much relevant information as possible in the shortest possible time. With practice, the history can be gleaned in a short time, but remember this is not the goal but comes with practice. Often in an effort to hurry, the examiner asks leading questions; this should be discouraged as it will lead to an inaccurate history. Most patients need help to describe their complaints and it is usually best to go through the history in chronological order. It is important to establish what the patient's immediate complaint is and the extent to which the symptoms are causing disability.

Pain is by far the commonest symptom, but the patient may complain more of the effect the pain has on his/her daily activities than of the pain itself. Symptoms other than pain may predominate. Joint stiffness or instability may be a problem and neurological disorders may result in characteristic functional difficulties. Many orthopaedic conditions are chronic and may result in the patient being unable to dress, manage normal toilet functions or go out of doors. The exact nature of the patient's work should be ascertained and

Lecture Notes: Orthopaedics and Fractures, 4e.
By T Duckworth and CM Blundell. Published 2010 by Blackwell Publishing.

some estimate should be made of how much working time is being lost because of illness. Financial worries may complicate the situation and may influence eventual decisions about treatment. It is helpful to get into the habit of making a provisional shortlist of possible diagnoses on the basis of the symptoms alone, as this helps to direct the history taking.

Pain

This is the commonest orthopaedic complaint. Its exact site should be determined and it should be remembered that referred pain is common, e.g. along the sciatic nerve from lesions in the lumbo-sacral spine, or into the arm from disease of the cervical spine.

The duration of the pain and its quality, e.g. aching, sharp, burning, etc, should be noted and also the degree to which it is aggravated by external factors such as walking or straining, as well as its response to analgesics. Pain is a *symptom* and is not the same as *tenderness*, which is a *physical sign*.

Stiffness

Stiffness of joints or inability to carry out a specific activity may also be a symptom, but it is surprisingly seldom that patients complain of this in the absence of pain.

Deformity or swelling

These may be the prevailing symptoms and it is important to ask the patient to point out, or describe, the abnormality. Where a swelling may be due to a neoplasm, the duration of symptoms can be all-important and the patient should be asked if the swelling has increased or fluctuated in size.

Weakness

This or similar loss of function may suggest a neurological abnormality. A full and detailed neurological history will then be required. Many neurological conditions present as disturbances of musculoskeletal function and many orthopaedic conditions may, in turn, produce neurological loss.

As a routine, enquiry should always be made as to whether there is any history of trauma, and details of previous surgical or other treatment should be sought. The history should always end with a general systematic enquiry which need only take a few seconds.

Examination

Much can be learnt from the patient's general appearance—does he/she look well or ill, haggard, wasted, feverish, etc? Does he/she appear nervous or over-anxious? Are his/her movements normal or is there a general or local abnormality of gait or in the use of arms and hands? Height, weight and build may be relevant, and in children, abnormalities of growth and development need to be considered, with due regard to the normal range of variation at any given age.

Local examination

The patient is more likely to feel at ease if the initial examination is directed to the part of the body of which he/she complains. A suggested scheme of examination is given below. *Both limbs should always be compared.*

Inspection

Attitude of the trunk and limbs

This includes the gait and stance. The patient should be watched as he/she walks, climbs on the examination couch, crouches or kneels, and uses his/her arms and hands. With practice, inspection of the gait may give a useful clue to the underlying disorder. It is usually easy to decide if the problem lies with the hip, knee or foot. Typical examples of common gait abnormalities include the Trendelenberg or 'dipping hip' gait, the stiff-legged gait of knee disease, and the gait associated with a painful foot, where the patient looks as though he/she is walking on hard pebbles. Many neurological disorders produce characteristic gait abnormalities, such as the tendency to 'back-knee' because of quadriceps weakness, or to catch the toe of the shoe as a result of a 'drop foot' gait associated with weakness of the ankle dorsiflexors.

Wasting

Localized or generalized muscle wasting may be an important and sometimes the only physical sign. It should always be searched for specifically and may not always be obvious when the patient is lying down.

Surface abnormalities

The whole skin surface should be inspected carefully for discoloration, scars, ulceration, bruising, rashes, etc.

Abnormalities of contour

The shape of the limb should be inspected for swelling, deformities, hollows, etc.

Palpation

Certain important physical signs can be elicited only by careful palpation. The whole area should be lightly but firmly palpated, and then attention directed to certain key diagnostic points.

Landmarks

A limb or joint may be grossly distorted by trauma or disease, and palpation should always begin by identifying the characteristic bony landmarks of the part, e.g. the anterior superior spine, greater trochanter, ischial tuberosity and symphysis pubis for the hip; for the elbow, the two epicondyles and the olecranon. The relationships between them should be carefully considered.

Tenderness

This is frequently the most important physical sign and must be localized accurately, e.g. is it maximal over the shaft, epiphysis, joint line, muscle, tendon, etc? It should be remembered that certain anatomical sites are quite tender in normal circumstances and it is always advisable to compare sides carefully.

Temperature

Comparison with the normal side is necessary and discrepancies caused by clothing or dressings must be avoided. Minor differences of temperature are more easily distinguished by palpating with the back of the hand.

Swelling

Any swelling must be carefully palpated and a note made of its size, position, shape, consistency, fluctuation, etc. Its position in relation to the various tissue planes and its attachments are particularly important. Is it attached to bone, muscle, tendon, skin, etc?

Movements

The main function of a joint is to allow movement, so that disturbances of movement are a usual accompaniment of joint disease.

Normal movements (i.e. within the normal planes)

Active movements

The patient should be asked to move the joint and the range of movements noted. In assessing joint ranges the anatomical position is usually taken as the reference point of 0 degrees (Fig. 15.1).

Passive movements

The examiner attempts to put the joint through a range of movements and notes the range and quality of the movements, i.e. is it smooth and progressive, or rough and crepitant, or is there a 'catch' at some point in the range? Occasionally the range is increased beyond the normal.

Abnormal movements

Joints rely for their stability mainly on ligaments, aided by muscle activity. When a ligament is ruptured it may be possible to move a joint in an abnormal direction. These movements should be tested specifically. Muscle relaxation is always essential for accurate ligament testing. An acute strain is likely to cause pain in the ligament when the latter is put on the stretch. Occasionally, an acute ligament rupture may have to be diagnosed by passively stressing the joint under X-ray control with local or general anaesthesia.

Causes of restriction of movements include:

1 Mechanical block, e.g. loose body, torn meniscus, etc
2 Soft-tissue contracture
3 Effusion
4 Paralysis
5 Spasm (and pain)
6 Spasticity.

Definition of deformity

The word is used in two senses:

1 Deformity of a bone means the bone is of abnormal shape or length, e.g. following a malunited fracture.
2 Deformity of a joint means that the joint *cannot be put into the anatomical position*. The deformity is named according to the direction in which the joint is bent, e.g. flexion deformity, adduction deformity, etc (Fig. 15.2). The word 'contracture' is often used in the same sense as deformity. A deformity essentially means a loss of range, but the converse is not necessarily true. The expression 'flexible deformity' is to some extent a contradiction in terms, but is used in the situation where the joint is held constantly in a deformed position, but can, in the appropriate circumstances, be put into the anatomical position. This is commonly the case with spastic conditions such as cerebral palsy, or following a stroke.

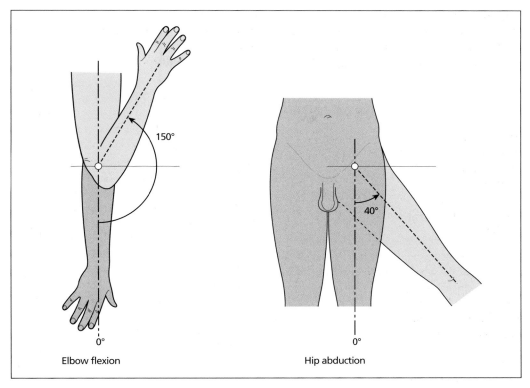

Figure 15.1 Joint range.

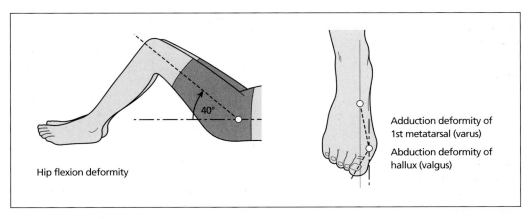

Figure 15.2 Joint deformities.

Measurements

Limb girth may be important in the assessment of wasting or swelling. The girth should always be compared with the normal side at a fixed distance from a bony landmark. Limb length may be measured as required, using a tape measure and again measuring between recognizable bony landmarks. It is difficult to achieve an accuracy of more than 1 cm.

Table 15.1 MRC scale for recording muscle power.

0	No muscle power
1	Flicker of activity
2	Movement with effect of gravity eliminated, i.e. in a plane at right angles to gravity but not against resistance
3	Movement against gravity but not against applied resistance
4	Movement against applied resistance but less than full power
5	Normal power

Table 15.2 Examination steps.

1	Inspection	Look
2	Palpation	Feel
3	Movement (active and passive)	Move
4	Measurement	
5	Neurology (motor/sensory)	
6	Circulation	Pulses
7	Lymphatics	Nodes

Neurological system

Many orthopaedic conditions are associated with neurological problems, and examination of the musculoskeletal system should *always* include a quick neurological assessment, which may be made more detailed if any abnormality is suspected.

The main points to be tested are:

1 Muscle power using the Medical Research Council (MRC) grading scale (Table 15.1) where relevant
2 Sensitivity to pinprick and cotton wool and
3 Reflexes.

Circulation

The colour and state of the limbs should be observed and pulses palpated. The presence or absence of hairs on the digits is often a useful test of circulatory insufficiency.

Both neurological and circulatory examinations are particularly important in assessing the injured limb.

Lymphatics

Where relevant, the lymphatic channels and nodes should be inspected and palpated. This is particularly important with tumours and acute infections.

Extent of examination

The above scheme can be applied to any part of the musculoskeletal system, but each area may require one or more specific tests which do not apply generally.

When examining a limb, it is usually necessary to split up movements and concentrate on each joint in turn. To examine the foot, for example, it is best to examine first the ankle, then the subtalar and mid-tarsal joints, then the forefoot and finally the toes.

The examination should, at the very least, include an assessment of all possible sources of disease relevant to the complaint; an examination of the abdomen and breasts should, for example, be considered routine for anyone complaining of low back pain; and pain in the hand normally warrants an examination of the neck.

If a careful history is taken and the examination is carried out as described above, it should be possible to arrive at a shortlist of differential diagnoses. It must, however, be admitted that in clinical practice many conditions are diagnosed on the basis of past experience—with the clinician employing a process of pattern recognition leading to a 'spot-diagnosis'.

The important steps in an orthopaedic examination are summarized in Table 15.2.

Part 2

Regional Orthopaedics

Chapter 16

The forearm, wrist and hand

The forearm

The upper end of the radius is a component of two joints—the elbow joint, where it contributes to the hinge mechanism, and the proximal radioulnar joint, where it provides for pronation and supination.

Both the hinge movements of the elbow and rotation of the forearm are usually still possible when the radial head is excised, but some stability to the varus and valgus stressing of the elbow is lost. Stability of the distal radioulnar joint depends on the integrity of the triangular fibro-cartilage attached to the ulnar styloid process. This structure is also a component of the wrist joint.

The wrist

The wrist joint proper is the articulation between the distal surface of the radius, the triangular fibro-cartilage and the proximal row of carpal bones—scaphoid, lunate and triquetrum (Fig. 16.1). This joint allows palmar and dorsiflexion and ulnar and radial deviation.

Further palmar and dorsiflexion is permitted at the joints between the proximal and distal rows of carpal bones. The metacarpals of the fingers,

Lecture Notes: Orthopaedics and Fractures, 4e.
By T Duckworth and CM Blundell. Published 2010 by Blackwell Publishing.

with the exception of the fifth, move very little at their bases, but the thumb metacarpal, which articulates only with the trapezium, has a considerable range.

The metacarpophalangeal joints (MCPJs) of the fingers allow considerable abduction and adduction in addition to flexion and extension, but the interphalangeal joints are simple hinge joints, with a collateral ligament on each side.

Examination of the forearm, wrist and hand (Box 16.1)

1 Inspection. Deformities should be noted; examples include the 'dinner fork' deformity of a Colles' fracture, and the 'mallet' or 'boutonnière' deformities of the fingers. Ulnar deviation of the fingers at the MCPJs is a manifestation of rheumatoid arthritis.

Wasting of individual muscle groups may be one of the first signs of neurological loss, e.g. the wasting of the thenar muscles in median nerve compression. Wasting of the interosseous muscles, best seen in the first dorsal interosseous muscle between thumb and index finger, may indicate an ulnar nerve lesion (Fig. 16.2).

Swellings are common in the wrist and hand; their extent and exact position in relation to the surrounding tissues should be determined. A high proportion of cystic swellings around the wrist are ganglia and these usually transilluminate.

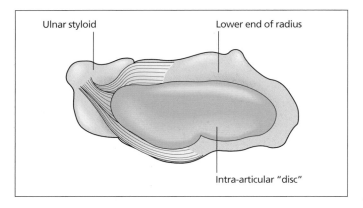

Ulnar styloid   Lower end of radius

Intra-articular "disc"

Figure 16.1 Proximal surface of wrist joint.

Box 16.1 Examination summary for hand, wrist and forearm.

Look	Deformity
	Wasting
	Swelling
Feel	Tenderness
	Temperature
	Transilluminate swelling
Move	Pronation/supination
	Dorsiflexion/palmar flexion

2 Palpation. Landmarks at the wrist are the styloid processes of the radius and ulna, the former normally lying more distally than the latter. The pisiform on the ulnar side and the scaphoid tubercle at the base of the thumb define the medial and lateral limits of the carpal tunnel.

Tenderness should be elicited carefully, and its exact position noted in relation to joints, ligaments, bones, tendons, etc.

Increased temperature is usual in infections of the hand and fingers. In these conditions oedema is common and this normally collects on the dorsum of the hand, even when the infection is in the palm.

3 Movements. The range of pronation and supination is usually measured from the mid-prone position, taking this as 0 degrees, rather than the anatomical position of full supination. Rotation through 90 degrees is usually possible in both directions. Wrist flexion and extension varies con-

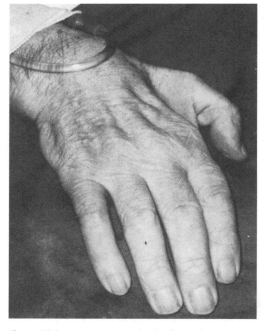

Figure 16.2 Intraosseous wasting in ulnar palsy.

siderably between individuals. Approximately 90 degrees in both directions is normal. Dorsiflexion can be easily compared on the two sides by asking the patient to place his/her palms together in a 'praying' position and then to elevate the elbows. Palmar flexion is similarly tested by placing the back of the hands together and dropping the elbows (Fig. 16.3). Radial and ulnar deviation is usually about 20 degrees, ulnar deviation being slightly greater.

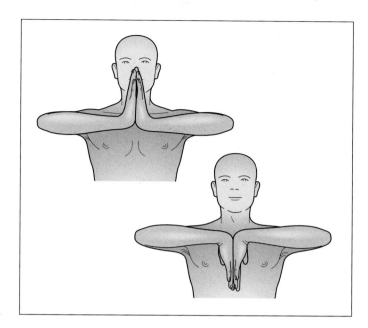

Figure 16.3 Testing wrist movements.

At the MCPJs, the range of flexion increases slightly from index to little finger. The range of flexion at the thumb MCPJ varies considerably from individual to individual, from a few degrees to 90 degrees (always compare both sides if pathology is suspected). The proximal interphalangeal joints of the fingers flex somewhat beyond 90 degrees, and the distal joints somewhat less than 90 degrees. Movements of the thumb relative to the palm is difficult to classify, but movement of the first metacarpal in a plane at right angles to the palm is usually called abduction and adduction, and movement in the plane at right angles to this is called flexion and extension. Internal rotation movement of the metacarpal is described as opposition. This classification corresponds to the names of the various muscles moving the thumb.

4 Measurement of the forearm is rarely helpful except in assessing muscle wasting.

5 Neurological examination.

6 Motor function. The functions of the hand and fingers are complex, and muscle groups and individual muscles should be tested systematically. A knowledge of the normal anatomy and physiology is essential. The following rules are helpful.

- Pronation is produced mainly by the pronator quadratus and pronator teres muscles (median nerve, C6, 7). Supination is a stronger movement produced principally by the biceps and supinator muscles (musculocutaneous and posterior interosseous nerves, C5, 6).
- The wrist flexors can be tested by asking the patient to flex the wrist and palpating the radial and ulnar flexor tendons (radialis, median nerve, C6, 7; ulnaris, ulnar nerve, C8, T1).
- All joints of the fingers are flexed by flexor digitorum profundus (median nerve to index and middle fingers, ulnar nerve to ring and little, C8, T1). Apart from the index, the profundus cannot flex individual fingers when the others are held extended. It is tested by asking the patient to flex the terminal interphalangeal joint whilst the proximal interphalangeal joint is held extended.
- The proximal interphalangeal joints are flexed by the flexor digitorum superficialis (sublimis) (median nerve, C7, 8, T1). It is tested by holding the other fingers extended and asking the patient to flex the appropriate finger.

• The MCPJs are normally flexed by the lumbrical and interosseous muscles. These also, through the dorsal expansions, extend the interphalangeal joints ('threading a needle' position). When these muscles are paralysed by an ulnar nerve lesion, the fingers take up a 'claw' position. Clawing of the index and middle fingers is less than the ring and little fingers because the lumbricals to these fingers are supplied by the median nerve (Fig. 16.4). The interossei are best tested by asking the patient to spread the fingers or to hold them tightly together. The hands can be compared by pressing the two little fingers together sideways (Fig. 16.5).

• The MCPJs are extended by the extensor digitorum longus, which can also extend the interphalangeal joints (posterior interosseous nerve, C7, 8).

• The thumb is flexed by the flexor pollicis longus (median nerve, C8, T1). The extensor pollicis longus extends the interphalangeal joint, and the extensor pollicis brevis extends the MCPJ and the carpometacarpal joint (posterior interosseous nerve, C7, 8).

• The thumb is abducted by the abductors pollicis brevis (median nerve, C8, T1) and longus (posterior interosseous nerve, C7, 8): adduction of the thumb and opposition by the thenar

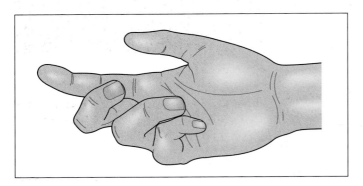

Figure 16.4 Ulnar palsy.

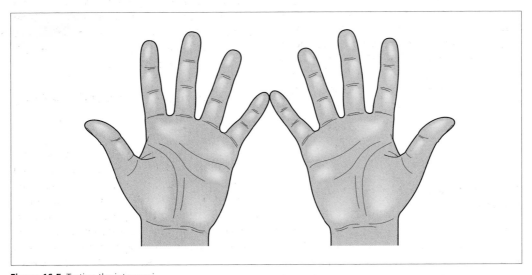

Figure 16.5 Testing the interossei.

group (median nerve, C8, T1) and the adductor pollicis (ulnar nerve, C8, T1).

• Wrist extension is produced by the extensor carpi ulnaris (posterior interosseous nerve, C7, 8), and extensor carpi radialis longus and brevis (posterior inter-osseous nerve, C6, 7).

7 Sensation. The dermatomes are as shown in the Appendix. Testing with a pin is adequate for most clinical purposes. In some circumstances, testing of two-point discrimination using dividers is a helpful test of fingertip sensory function.

8 Circulation. The radial pulse is easily palpable. The integrity of the radial and ulnar arteries can be determined using Allen's test.

9 Lymphatic system. Lymphangitis and lymph gland enlargement are common in hand and finger infections.

Developmental conditions

1 Madelung's deformity. This is a complex deformity of the distal end of the radius. Due to a growth defect of the radius, the lower end of the ulna becomes prominent.

2 Multiple enchondromatosis (see p. 67 and Fig. 9.2) usually causes multiple swellings in the digits, often with considerable interference with function. Repeated surgery may be necessary over a long period. Achondroplasia produces a hand with short fingers and often a single transverse palmar crease.

3 Trigger thumb. This common condition most often affects the thumbs of babies. Constriction of the flexor tendon sheath opposite the the metacarpal head results in a flexed interphalangeal joint. A nodule can often be felt at the site of constriction. Longitudinal division of the tendon sheath is curative.

Traumatic conditions

Fracture of the shafts of the radius and ulna

These are common injuries. An isolated displaced fracture of the mid-shaft of either bone can occur if either the radial head subluxates with an ulnar fracture (Monteggia fracture; Fig. 16.6) or the lower

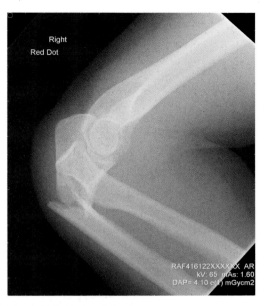

Figure 16.6 Monteggia fracture.

end of the ulna subluxates with a fracture of the radius (Galeazzi fracture; Fig. 16.7). Fractures of both bones are more usual.

Treatment

Accurate alignment is essential for all these shaft fractures to allow pronation and supination. They are usually treated by open reduction and plating. Greenstick fractures in children may be manipulated and held in a plaster-cast, which must include the wrist and the elbow, bent to 90 degrees, to control rotation of the forearm.

Fracture of the distal end of the radius

Colles' fracture

The term has come to mean a fracture within 1 inch of the distal end of the radius and is one of the commonest fractures of middle and old age. There is dorsal tilt, dorsal displacement and, often, impaction of the distal fragment, producing shortening of the radius and radial deviation of the wrist (Fig. 16.8). The fracture may be comminuted as the bone is frequently osteoporotic. The styloid process of the ulna is often avulsed.

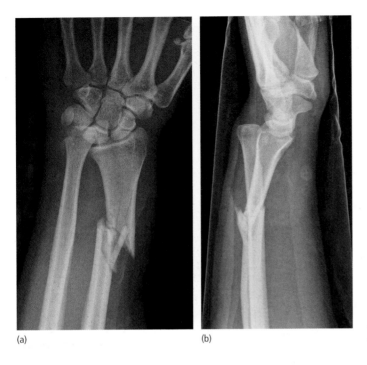

(a)   (b)

Figure 16.7 (a) AP X-ray of Galleazzi fracture; **(b)** lateral X-ray of Galleazzi fracture—note displacement of ulna.

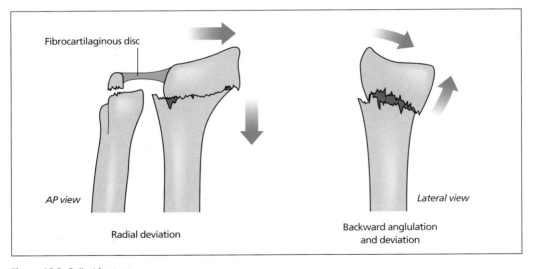

Figure 16.8 Colles' fracture.

A Colles' fracture is almost always produced by a fall on the outstretched hand. It produces a characteristic 'dinner fork' deformity of the forearm and wrist (Fig. 16.9).

Complications

Median nerve symptoms are not uncommon, but usually subside after reduction. Median nerve compression also occurs occasionally as a late complication of a badly reduced fracture. Malunion may be associated with pain from a subluxated distal radioulnar joint, the pain tending to occur on rotation of the forearm. Distal radial fractures may also be complicated by a rupture of a tendon crossing the fracture line, such as the extensor pollicis longus. Complex regional pain syndrome is a rare complication (see p. 45).

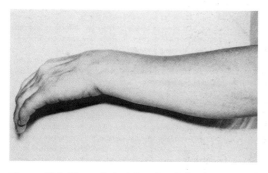

Figure 16.9 Dinner fork deformity of the forearm and wrist.

Treatment

If the fracture is only minimally displaced, reduction is not necessary. A useful way of assessing the need for reduction is to draw a line between the two lips of the articular surface of the radius on the lateral film. If this line is at right angles or slightly tilted forwards relative to the line of the radial shaft, then reduction is not necessary. Any backward tilt of this line suggests the need for reduction (Fig. 16.10).

The usual method of reducing the fracture is by manipulation under anaesthesia.

A dorsal plaster slab is prepared, of a size sufficient to cover the forearm and wrist to the level of the knuckles and to extend around the sides of the forearm, but not to meet at the front. The elbow is held by an assistant and traction is applied to disimpact the distal fragment, which is then flexed, pushed in a palmar direction and towards the ulnar side. Keeping traction on the thumb in line with the forearm, the slab is applied to a layer of wool applied over the dorsal aspect of the wrist and

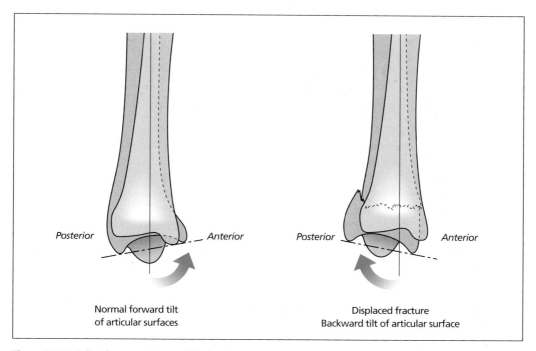

Normal forward tilt of articular surfaces

Displaced fracture
Backward tilt of articular surface

Figure 16.10 Colles' fracture—degree of displacement.

forearm. The wrist is held in slight flexion and in slight ulnar deviation. The slab is held in place with a gauze bandage and, whilst the plaster is setting, the fracture is moulded using the ball of the thumb. A check X-ray is then taken and, if all is well, the arm is supported in a sling. Swelling is usual, but subsides with use of the hand. It is important to instruct the patient to exercise the fingers, the elbow and the shoulder. It is usual to see the patient next day to check the cast and again 1 week later when an X-ray is taken to check that the position has not been lost. The plaster may then be completed. The cast is removed at 5–6 weeks and exercises started if the tenderness has almost disappeared, as is usual.

In the child, the fracture is usually of the greenstick type and reduction is rarely necessary. Two or 3 weeks in a plaster slab is sufficient to allow healing to occur.

Smith's fracture

This is a fracture of the lower end of the radius with palmar angulation.

Treatment
Smith's fracture is usually treated by open reduction and internal fixation with a plate applied to the palmar aspect of the radius.

Slipped lower radial epiphysis

This injury is similar to a Colles' fracture, but occurring through the epiphyseal line in a child. It is usually Type II in the Salter and Harris classification (see p. 28). It is easy to manipulate if this is done within the first 3 days and 3 weeks' immobilization in a plaster back slab is sufficient.

Fractures of the scaphoid

This injury usually occurs in working men as a result of a blow to the palm of the hand or a fall on the hand.

Diagnosis
This is partly clinical and partly radiological, the main physical signs being swelling and tenderness in the 'anatomical snuff box' with pain on wrist movements and on longitudinal compression of the thumb. In addition to the usual AP and lateral views, oblique or 'scaphoid' views of the wrist are necessary. It is usually suggested that if the clinical signs suggest a fracture, but the X-ray is negative, the wrist should be immobilized for 2 weeks, then re-X-rayed, when the fracture will often be revealed if present.

Complications
Fractures through the waist may deprive the proximal half of the bone of its blood. When this occurs, union becomes uncertain and avascular necrosis of the proximal fragment may occur (Fig. 16.11).

Treatment
The wrist is immobilized in a plaster in the neutral position, the plaster extending from the elbow to the MCPJs. If the thumb is included, this is termed a 'scaphoid' plaster (Fig. 16.12). Immobilization

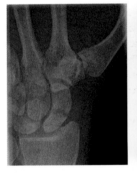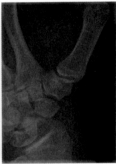

Figure 16.11 Fracture of the scaphoid—avascular necrosis.

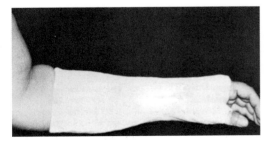

Figure 16.12 Scaphoid plaster-cast.

must be continued until the clinical signs disappear and there is radiological evidence of union. This takes at least 6 weeks and may take several months.

Sometimes the fracture fails to unite as a result of damage to the blood supply or displacement of the fracture. Symptomatic non-union necessitates surgery, but it is worth remembering that many non-unions are relatively symptom-free, and indeed may only be discovered accidentally when the wrist is X-rayed for some other reason. Non-union of a scaphoid fracture is most frequently treated with a bone graft and a screw across the fracture line. A useful screw for this purpose has been devised by Herbert. It has threads on each end which are of different pitches, so that when tightened it compresses the fragments together. In some units internal fixation is used to treat acute fractures. Screw fixation is used when the fracture is associated with a dislocation of the wrist.

Dislocations of the carpus

These are uncommon injuries and are often missed. Sometimes there is no fracture and the lunate is left *in situ* whilst the rest of the carpus dislocates—a perilunate dislocation. On occasions, the scaphoid fractures through the waist and, when displacement occurs, the proximal pole of the scaphoid and the whole of the lunate are left behind: a transscaphoid–perilunate dislocation (Fig. 16.13).

Complications
Median nerve compression commonly accompanies these injuries.

Treatment
This is initially by manipulation, followed by operative repair and immobilization in a cast for approximately 6 weeks. In a transscaphoid–perilunate dislocation, internal fixation of the scaphoid is usually advisable.

Bennett's fracture

This is a fracture dislocation of the carpometacarpal joint of the thumb. It is usually treated by closed reduction and a percutaneous Kirschner wire to stabilize the carpometacarpal joint (Fig. 16.14). Four weeks in plaster is usually sufficient for union.

Fractures of the metacarpals

These are common injuries. It is important that these fractures do not unite with malrotation because this affects the plane of finger flexion. Spiral fractures, particularly, may require internal fixation to avoid this complication. A fracture of the neck of the fifth metacarpal often follows a blow with the fist ('boxer's fracture'). The majority of these injuries do not require manipulation and heal within 3 weeks with simple strapping.

Fractures of the phalanges

These injuries can be difficult to treat. They may be open and associated with tendon and nerve damage.

Treatment
Simple fractures of the phalanges can often be treated by strapping the finger to the adjacent one, known as neighbour strapping, which helps to control rotation. If manipulation is required, the reduction can usually be maintained by strapping the injured finger to a malleable splint.

The more difficult fractures, especially at the ends of the bones, may need open reduction and fixation with Kirschner wires or small plates.

Fractures of the terminal phalanges are caused by crush injuries. They are often open injuries and associated with damage to the nailbed.

Partial amputation of the tip may be treated by a skin flap (Fig. 16.15). It is often simpler to carry out a partial amputation of the phalanx to allow skin to be fashioned to cover the finger end.

Mallet finger

This is an avulsion injury of the extensor tendon from the base of the terminal phalanx (Fig. 16.16).

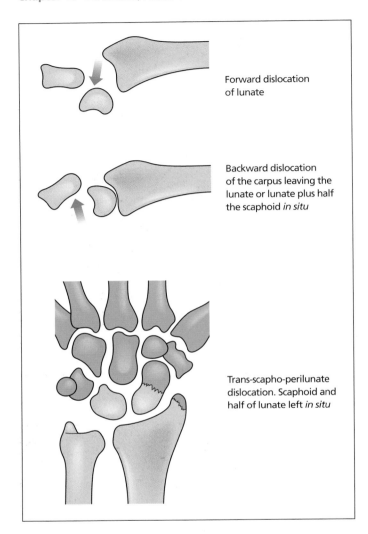

Forward dislocation of lunate

Backward dislocation of the carpus leaving the lunate or lunate plus half the scaphoid *in situ*

Trans-scapho-perilunate dislocation. Scaphoid and half of lunate left *in situ*

Figure 16.13 Dislocation/fracture of the wrist.

Treatment

It is possible to secure healing using a malleable splint to hyper-extend the terminal interphalangeal joint and allow flexion of the proximal interphalangeal joint (Fig. 16.17). Healing is more likely to occur if the tendon has avulsed a fragment of bone from the base of the phalanx. At least 6 weeks' splintage is usually necessary. Treatment is not always successful and the patient may be left with an 'extension lag', i.e. the inability to extend the terminal joint actively, even though passive extension is full. This is not usually troublesome. If the fingertip tends to 'get in the way', the interphalangeal joint may need fusion later.

Dislocations of the finger joints

These can usually be reduced easily and are reasonably stable. They are supported by strapping adjacent fingers together and movement is usually allowed immediately.

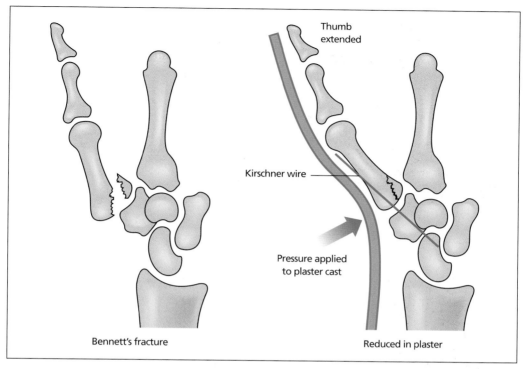

Thumb
extended

Kirschner wire

Pressure applied
to plaster cast

Bennett's fracture

Reduced in plaster

Figure 16.14 Bennett's fracture.

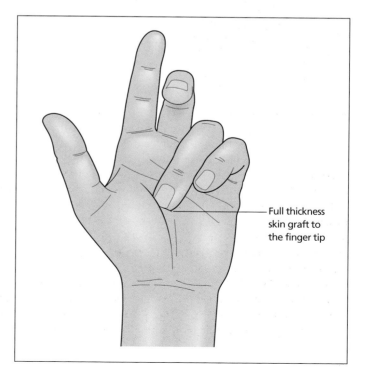

Full thickness
skin graft to
the finger tip

Figure 16.15 Full thickness skin graft
to the fingertip.

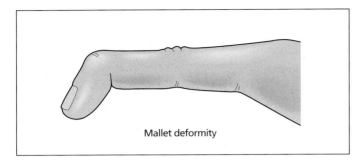

Mallet deformity

Figure 16.16 Mallet finger.

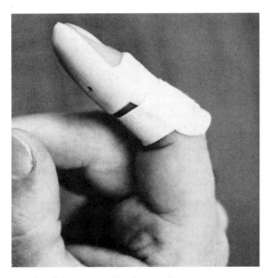

Figure 16.17 Plastic mallet finger splint.

> **Box 16.2** Key points in the management of hand injuries.
>
> - Amputation in severe injuries may be the best option
> - Preserve as much thumb as possible
> - An insensate digit is almost useless
> - Complex crush injuries are best managed in specialist centres with a hand service

plaster-cast. If the instability is obvious, surgical repair, followed by plaster immobilization is advisable.

Management of hand injuries (Box 16.2)

All these injuries, especially serious open ones, are prone to stiffness and treatment should be aimed at early movement and use of the hand as soon as possible.

Infective conditions

Acute infections (see Chapter 13)

1 **Acute paronychia**—infection under the nailfold.

2 **Apical abscess**—a small collection of pus under the end of a nail.

3 **Intradermal abscess**—a collection of pus on the palmar surface of the finger or hand, lying between the deep and superficial layers of the dermis, it may communicate with a second collection in the deep tissues—collar stud abscess (Fig. 16.18).

4 **Pulp space infection**—the pulp space of the finger is divided by septa and becomes very tense and painful if sepsis occurs. The phalanx (usually

Rupture of the ulnar collateral ligament of the thumb

Sometimes known as 'gamekeeper's' or 'skier's' thumb, the injury is a partial or complete rupture of the ulnar collateral ligament of the MCPJ and is caused by forced abduction. If it is unrecognized and allowed to heal with lengthening, it results in instability which interferes with the 'pinch' grip of the thumb against the index finger. It should be suspected if there is tenderness over the ligament and the instability may be demonstrable by comparing it with the opposite side.

Treatment

Minor degrees of instability, suggesting a strain or partial tear, may be treated in a scaphoid-type

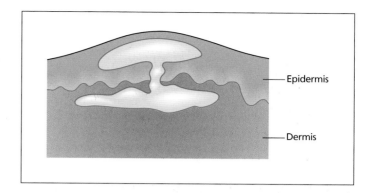

Figure 16.18 Collar stud abscess.

terminal) may become secondarily infected and an X-ray is essential if infection is well-established.

5 Web space infections—infection occurs between the fingers and pus may point in the web.

6 Deep palmar space infection—suppuration may be localized to one or other of the anatomical palmar spaces.

Treatment

Conditions 1–4 may respond to antibiotics in the early stages, but if pus has formed, surgical drainage is necessary. The acute paronychia is drained by an incision parallel to the nail edge or part of the nail is removed. The other conditions are drained by direct incision, avoiding sensitive areas if possible and conserving skin.

If osteomyelitis has occurred the infected bone may need to be excised.

Both web and palmar space infections cause gross swelling of the hand with oedema of the dorsum. Elevation, usually in hospital, and antibiotic therapy may avoid pus formation, but when pus is present or suspected, incision is necessary.

Suppurative tenosynovitis

This is a serious condition usually originating from a penetrating injury, which may be minor. The tendon sheath fills with fluid and later pus. Early diagnosis is important as the tendon may become adherent or even slough, and the infection may extend into the deep palm. The digit is swollen, very painful and tender along the whole length of the sheath. All movements are painful.

Treatment

Treatment is by elevation of the hand and drainage, usually through two incisions, one distally in the finger, either in the mid-lateral line or in the distal crease, and a second in the distal palm crease (Fig. 16.19). The sheath is then irrigated and intravenous antibiotics are administered. Primary healing is usual in the early case.

In all hand infections, resting the hand with the fingers and thumb in the functional resting position is important for ultimate function.

Neoplastic conditions

Metastatic tumours are relatively uncommon in the forearm and hand. Pain in this area may be referred from a bronchial neoplasm affecting the apex of the lung and invading the brachial plexus (Pancoast tumour).

Of the primary tumours, enchondromata arising in the fingers and usually expanding the digit are relatively common. Giant cell tumours occasionally arise in relation to the tendon sheaths. Lipomata and neurofibromata may occur singly or as part of a widespread syndrome. Other neoplasms are uncommon.

Metabolic disorders

Most of the metabolic disorders produce recognizable radiological abnormalities in the bones of the wrist and hand. Measurement of the density of the metacarpal is sometimes used as an index of the severity of osteoporosis ('metacarpal

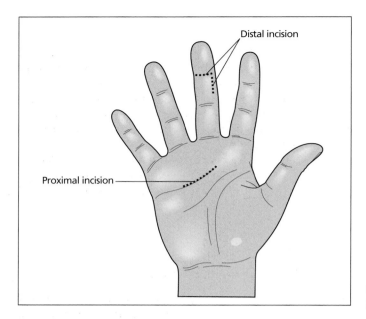

Figure 16.19 Incisions for draining a palmar space infection.

index'). Symptoms are, however, uncommon. Hyperparathyroidism may cause bone pain.

Paget's disease may affect the radius, but rarely the ulna, and may cause the bone to become elongated and curved. Bone pain is an occasional complaint but changes in the hands are rare.

Degenerative conditions

Pain in the forearm and hand, occasionally with neurology, may be the presenting feature of a cervical disc prolapse, cervical spondylosis or cervical rib. See also:

1 Carpal tunnel syndrome (see p. 20)
2 Tenosynovitis (see p. 90)
3 Ganglion (see p. 91).

De Quervain's tenovaginitis

This condition is due to thickening of the tendon sheaths of the abductor pollicis longus and extensor pollicis brevis where they cross the radial styloid. Repeated movements may be responsible for some cases.

Clinical features

The patient complains of pain at the site, made worse by gripping and by extending the thumb. Forced flexion of the thumb whilst the wrist is deviated to the ulnar side also causes pain. There is localized tenderness and often a swelling over the radial styloid.

Treatment

A hydrocortisone injection may give rapid relief. Alternatively a period of 2–3 weeks in a plastercast, including the thumb, may cure the condition. Resistant cases can be treated by opening the sheath surgically, making sure that all the tendinous strips are completely freed.

Trigger finger

This is a similar condition affecting the sheath of the flexor tendon and causing the tendon to stick as it passes under a tendon pulley. Alternatively, the patient may be unable to extend the finger actively from the fully flexed position. A nodule is usually palpable at the site of thickening, opposite the head of the metacarpal. The condition occurs occasionally in young babies, almost always affecting the thumb ('clasped thumb').

Treatment

The condition may resolve spontaneously. Steroid injections into the sheath may be effective, but if this fails, the condition can be readily cured by longitudinal division of the tendon pulley, ensuring that the tendon runs freely. Both trigger finger and De Quervain's tenovaginitis may be an early manifestation of rheumatoid arthritis.

Dupuytren's contracture

This is a condition affecting the collagenous tissue of the palmar fascia. There is frequently a family history. It is occasionally related to cirrhosis of the liver, diabetes and rarely to drugs used to treat epilepsy. It affects middle-aged men much more commonly than women.

Clinical features

1 The characteristic feature is a very slowly progressing flexion contracture of the fingers and thumb. It is usually bilateral but may be more severe on one side.
2 The palmar fascia feels thickened and nodular and tends to pucker the overlying skin. Definite bands can be felt running along the sides of the fingers due to thickening of the lateral extensions of the fascia.
3 The proximal interphalangeal joint is usually most affected, together with the MCPJ.
4 Thickened pads may develop over the knuckles and occasionally nodules may occur on the medial side of the sole of the foot.

Treatment

Usually, surgery is necessary for the established contracture with symptoms and this involves careful dissection of the whole of the affected area of fascia. Skin closure can be difficult but the skin usually heals well. Occasionally, the fascia is removed with the overlying skin (dermo-fasciectomy) and subsequently the area is covered with a free skin flap. Occasionally, a finger may be better amputated if deformity is very severe.

Osteoarthritis

Osteoarthritis may affect joints damaged by disease or injury, e.g. osteoarthritis of the wrist following a non-united fracture of the scaphoid.

Osteoarthritis of the joint between the trapezium and base of the first metacarpal is common. It may be treated, if severe enough, by excision of the trapezium.

Osteoarthritis of the terminal interphalangeal joints of the fingers (Heberden's nodes) is common and is usually a manifestation of generalized osteoarthritis.

Inflammatory conditions

Rheumatoid arthritis

Involvement of the joints and synovial sheaths of the hand is usual in this condition. Stiffness and swelling of the finger joints are frequently the presenting symptoms. As the disease progresses, the joints are gradually destroyed. Destruction of the articular surfaces and attenuation of the ligaments combine to produce the characteristic ulnar deviation of the fingers at the MCPJs.

Inflammatory involvement of the synovial sheaths, particularly of the extensor tendons, causes painful swelling and eventually may cause rupture of the tendons. Swan-neck and boutonnière deformities may occur (Fig. 16.20), but despite these various deformities and the associated pain and stiffness, function is often preserved for a surprisingly long period.

Treatment

Local measures include rest and splintage during the acute phases. Surgery can offer synovectomy of the tendon sheaths and joints, repair of ruptured tendons, and arthroplasties for the various involved joints. Several forms of arthroplasty for the finger joints are available, but a popular one is a flexible silastic implant devised by Swanson, which gives stability whilst still allowing movement. Arthrodesis of the wrist can also be helpful in relieving pain and maintaining function in the hand.

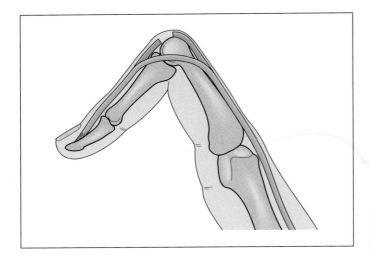

Figure 16.20 Rupture of the middle slip of the extensor tendon producing 'boutonnière' deformity.

Psoriasis

Severe involvement of the hands is unusual, but swelling of the tendon synovial sheaths and moderate involvement of the wrists does occur occasionally. Pitting of the nails may be a useful diagnostic sign.

Chapter 17

The elbow

The elbow is a stable joint which is prone to stiffness following injury, even when the injury is relatively minor.

Anatomy

The elbow joint functions as a simple hinge, its stability depending on the close fit of the trochlea in the trochlear notch of the ulna. The superior radioulnar joint functions as part of the hinge and also as the rotation point for pronation and supination of the forearm.

The epiphyseal centres of the lower humerus appear between the ages of 2 and 12 (Fig. 17.1). Fractures of the condyles in children often separate off much larger fragments than the X-ray appearances would suggest.

Examination

1 Inspection. Deformity should be noted. Flexion deformities are common and may follow even minor injuries. Trauma to the elbow may result in disturbance of growth on either side of the joint, causing cubitus valgus (increased carrying angle) or cubitus varus (decreased carrying angle). Increasing cubitus valgus carries the risk of ulnar

Lecture Notes: Orthopaedics and Fractures, 4e.
By T Duckworth and CM Blundell. Published 2010 by
Blackwell Publishing.

nerve damage due to traction (see p. 21). Wasting of the biceps and triceps is common in many elbow conditions.

2 Palpation. The bony landmarks are the olecranon and the two epicondyles. In the flexed position these form the points of an equilateral triangle, but when the arm is extended they lie on a straight line (Fig. 17.2). The radial head can be palpated below the lateral epicondyle and is often slightly tender in the normal individual.

3 Movements. The normal elbow range of flexion and extension is from 0 to 150 degrees. Pronation and supination are 90 degrees each from the mid position. Note that the mid-prone position rather than the anatomical position is usually taken as zero. It should not be possible to tilt the forearm medially or laterally in full extension. — N locked"

Congenital conditions

Congenital dislocation of the radial head occurs very rarely. Most often it is an anterior dislocation and may be associated with other congenital malformations. Treatment is rarely necessary, but occasionally removal of the radial head in early adult life may be helpful if motion is restricted.

Traumatic conditions

Injuries around and involving the elbow are very prone to result in stiffness and a long period of

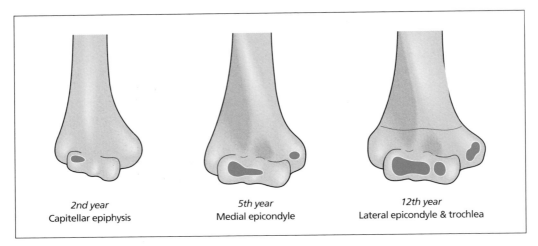

| 2nd year | 5th year | 12th year |
| Capitellar epiphysis | Medial epicondyle | Lateral epicondyle & trochlea |

Figure 17.1 Ossification centres at the elbow.

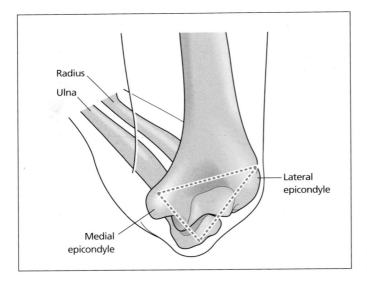

Radius
Ulna
Lateral epicondyle
Medial epicondyle

Figure 17.2 Relationship of the landmarks at the elbow.

mobilization may be necessary to regain full movements, even in children.

Dislocation of the elbow

This is usually produced by a fall on the hand with the elbow partially flexed.

Clinical features

The elbow is swollen and held in a flexed position. The ulna is displaced backwards on the lower end of the humerus (Fig. 17.3). The radial head may be fractured, as may the coronoid process.

Complications

Median nerve palsy occasionally occurs, but the prognosis for recovery is good. Brachial artery damage is rare.

Treatment

Reduction is usually easy, sometimes without anaesthesia. The operator, keeping the elbow·

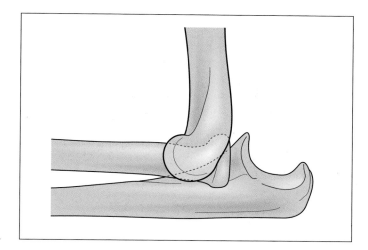

Figure 17.3 Dislocation of the elbow.

flexed, puts his/her fingers around the epicondyles from behind and pushes forwards on the olecranon with his/her thumbs. The elbow is then initially immobilized in a simple sling or collar and cuff and providing there are no fractures, the patient is permitted to mobilize the elbow as comfort allows.

Fracture dislocation of the elbow

This is usually a severe injury, e.g. the 'side-swipe' injury sustained by a blow to the elbow held hanging out of a car window. There may be fractures of the condyles of the humerus or the radial head or, most commonly, of the olecranon. In the worst injuries there may be multiple fractures.

Treatment
Manipulative reduction or internal fixation may be necessary, but a stiff elbow is the usual outcome. Attempts are usually made to stabilize the elbow so that early mobilization can be attempted. If it is completely detached or badly shattered, the radial head may need to be removed, but its absence increases the risk of instability. A prosthetic radial head replacement is available and should be used if, following removal of shattered radial head fragments, the elbow feels unstable.

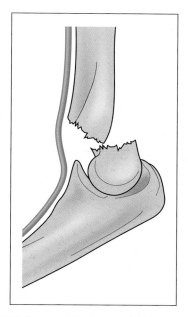

Figure 17.4 Supracondylar fracture of the humerus.

Supracondylar fracture of the humerus

This is essentially an injury occurring in childhood, usually arising from a fall on the outstretched hand. The lower fragment is typically displaced and rotated backwards (Fig. 17.4). The elbow usually swells considerably and is held in a semi-flexed position. Crepitus may be felt on attempting to move the joint.

Complications

The sharp anterior margin of the upper fragment may kink the brachial artery, which may also be injured if the elbow is flexed before reducing the fracture. The radial pulse may not be palpable, but usually the circulation remains adequate. Nerve injuries are uncommon but both median and ulnar palsies may occur. Late deformity occasionally occurs because of malunion ('gunstock' deformity).

Treatment

This is by manipulation under anaesthesia with X-ray control. The elbow is kept flexed to about 60 degrees and the epicondyles are held between the operator's fingers whilst the fragment is pulled downwards and forwards. The epicondyles must be kept level, otherwise the fracture may unite with a tilt. Having reduced the fracture and checked it on X-rays, holding the arm in a collar and cuff sling against the chest usually gives reasonably accurate rotation of the lower fragment on the upper. The elbow should not be flexed much above 90 degrees, particularly if swelling is severe, as this may impair the distal circulation.

Post-operative management

The patient is admitted and the circulation in the limb watched over the next 24 hours. The pulse may not return after manipulation, but this in itself is not a cause for alarm, provided the circulation remains adequate.

Pain in the forearm flexor region and particularly on passive extension of the fingers is a warning sign of ischaemia of the forearm muscles. If this is untreated it will result in muscle necrosis and later contracture of the fingers, known as Volkmann's ischaemic contracture. ← fibrosis

If the circulation is not restored by extending the elbow, the artery should be explored and if damaged, a segment may need to be resected and grafted.

Occasionally, the fracture is unstable in the flexed position and traction (Fig. 17.5) or even immobilization in extension may be necessary. If instability is difficult to control by an external technique, internal fixation may be the best option. The position can usually be held with two Kirschner wires driven across the fracture line from the lateral side of the distal fragment, taking great care not to damage the ulnar nerve. The wires are removed after 3 weeks.

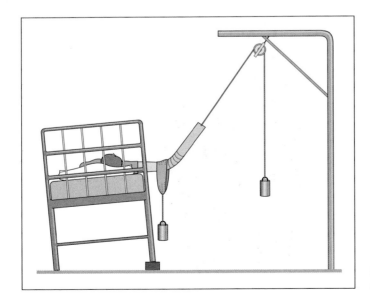

Figure 17.5 Dunlop traction for supracondylar fracture.

Fractures of the epicondyles

These injuries usually occur in children from a fall on the arm.

Medial epicondyle

The medial epicondyle may be avulsed by the medial ligament (Fig. 17.6), and when this happens it occasionally becomes trapped in the medial side of the elbow joint and is visible there on a lateral X-ray film (Fig. 17.7).

Treatment

Manipulation may be possible by abducting the elbow and attempting to draw out the fragment by extending the wrist and fingers. If this fails, surgery is necessary to extract the fragment from the joint and reposition it. It may be stable in its normal position or it may need to be pinned.

Lateral condyle

A fracture of the lateral condyle in a child involves a much larger piece of bone than is obvious on X-ray (Fig. 17.8).

Treatment

The fragment usually needs pinning back in position to avoid non-union and later deformity due to interference with the growing epiphysis. In particular, cubitus valgus may occur and this is often associated with ulnar palsy later in life (p. 20).

Intercondylar or T-shaped fracture of the humerus

This usually occurs in adults, as a combination of a supracondylar fracture and a vertical break between the two condyles.

Treatment

This normally involves open reduction and rigid internal fixation. Providing this can be achieved early, mobilization of the elbow can be permitted, which reduces the risk of post-operative joint stiffness.

Fracture of the radial head

These are essentially produced by abduction injuries in which the head is driven against the capitulum, and the medial ligament is strained.

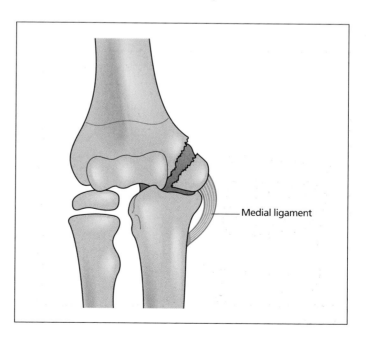

Figure 17.6 Fracture of the medial epicondyle.

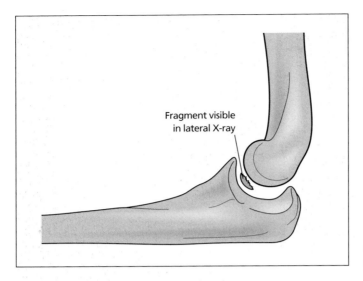

Fragment visible
in lateral X-ray

Figure 17.7 Trapped bone fragment with fracture of the medial epicondyle.

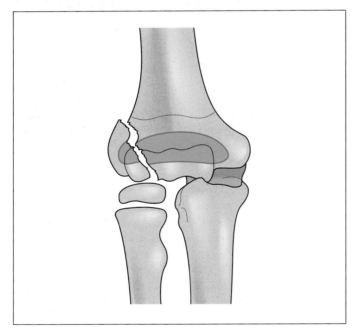

Figure 17.8 The ossified epiphysis visible on the X-ray is only a small part of a large fragment.

Clinical features

The elbow is swollen and painful and there is localized tenderness over the radial head and also usually on the medial side. All movements are restricted and pain is usually experienced on pronation and supination. Diagnosis is confirmed on the X-ray features (Fig. 17.9).

Treatment

Minor cracks and undisplaced fractures may be supported in a sling and mobilized early. Comminuted fractures may restrict rotation and are best treated by excision of the radial head at the earliest opportunity. It is helpful, in deciding whether to excise the head, to check the range of

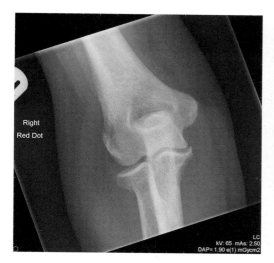

Figure 17.9 Fracture of the radial head.

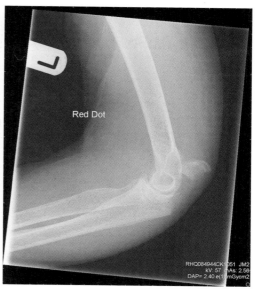

Figure 17.10 Fracture of the olecranon.

pronation and supination. If this range is good, it is reasonable to leave the head *in situ* and concentrate on mobilizing the elbow.

Single head fragments, if large enough, may be suitable for open reduction and fixation with a tiny screw or wire. With severe comminution, the radius may move upwards, causing subluxation of the inferior radioulnar joint. In these circumstances, a radial head prosthesis is necessary to restore joint alignment.

In the child, the radial head represents the epiphysis and may be displaced and tilted. It is often possible to correct this by manipulation and it is then reasonably stable. Open reduction is occasionally needed, but again the fracture is usually stable after reduction. The head should not be excised.

Pulled elbow

This is an injury of young children who have been pulled forcibly by the arm. It is caused by the radial head slipping out of the annular ligament, and is usually easily treated by simply rotating the elbow and allowing the radial head to click back into position—a click may be felt once only as the head reduces.

Fracture of the olecranon

These may occur as part of a fracture dislocation of the elbow (see Fig. 16.6, p.127), or as an isolated injury. The proximal fragment is usually pulled away from the distal fragment by the triceps muscle (Fig. 17.10).

Treatment

In an elderly patient, the position may be accepted and the elbow mobilized in the hope of avoiding stiffness. There will usually be some residual weakness of extension, e.g. when reaching up to a shelf above shoulder height.

In all other patients, open reduction and internal fixation using a long screw or tension-band technique gives the best results and almost full movements may be achieved (see Fig. 5.13).

Infection

Osteomyelitis

This occasionally affects the lower end of the humerus or upper end of the radius and ulna. Suppurative arthritis is uncommon in the elbow except in association with rheumatoid arthritis.

145

Chronic infections

Tuberculosis of the elbow is rare, though it is increasing in incidence. It is usually associated with considerable muscular wasting. If ankylosis seems inevitable, splintage in a functional position is necessary. In a right-handed person, flexion of at least 90 degrees is necessary in the right elbow to enable the patient to feed easily. If both elbows are stiff, one should be fixed at just over 90 degrees and the other at 20–30 degrees to enable toilet functions to be performed.

Neoplastic conditions

Metastases may occur in any of the bones around the elbow, but primary tumours are rare.

Degenerative conditions

Tennis elbow

This is a very common condition which was originally described in lawn tennis players. It affects people whose work involves a lot of gripping and twisting of the forearm, such as car mechanics and bricklayers. It is thought to be a degenerative condition, but there is little pathological evidence for this. There have also been suggestions that the condition may be due to a localized entrapment of the radial or posterior interosseous nerve, but the evidence for this is unconvincing.

Clinical features
The condition affects the origin of the extensor muscles of the wrist, particularly the extensor carpi radialis brevis, and typically causes chronic pain on the outer side of the elbow radiating down the outer border of the forearm, especially when gripping. Tenderness is accurately localized over the front of the lateral epicondyle. Extending the elbow and simultaneously pronating the forearm and flexing the wrist and fingers exacerbates the pain. There are no X-ray changes.

Management
The condition almost always settles spontaneously, but may last many months. Rest and local hydrocortisone injections relieve symptoms in about 70% of patients. Rarely, surgery may be indicated, with detachment of the whole or part of the common extensor origin from the lateral epicondyle.

Golfer's elbow

This is a very similar condition to tennis below, but it affects the medial side, with tenderness over the medial epicondyle and pain on hyper-extending the fingers and wrist.

Olecranon bursitis

Acute

This usually occurs in people whose occupation involves leaning on the elbows. The bursa becomes acutely swollen and inflamed. Rarely, the bursa is infected and fills with pus.

Treatment
Aspiration may be necessary if the bursa is very tense. If pus is aspirated, drainage and antibiotic therapy is indicated.

Chronic

The bursa is chronically distended with fluid and there is a tendency for the exudate, which contains fibrin, to form small nodules or 'melon-seed bodies'. These are usually tender, but pain is not usually a prominent feature of chronic olecranon bursitis.

Treatment
Aspiration drains straw-coloured fluid which is not infected. This rarely cures the condition and excision of the bursa may be necessary if it continues to cause symptoms.

Osteochondritis dissecans

The bony fragment may separate from the capitulum or trochlea and become free as a loose body, causing intermittent pain, locking and swelling.

The condition is often bilateral and may go undiagnosed until osteoarthritis supervenes later in life.

Osteoarthritis

The elbow not infrequently becomes osteoarthritic, particularly in those doing manual work. Symptoms may involve aching discomfort or acute pain due to locking of the elbow as a result of loose bodies. Often, however, the patient notices only a lack of full extension of the elbow. The patient is usually male and in his 40s or 50s.

Treatment

Conservative treatment is usually adequate. Occasionally excision of loose bodies or the radial head may be helpful.

Inflammatory conditions

The elbow is frequently affected by rheumatoid arthritis. The joint is gradually destroyed and may become unstable. All the joint surfaces are affected, particularly the humeroradial.

Clinical features

Pain and swelling are usual features, with synovial thickening and often a considerable effusion. Stiffness is not usually severe and more commonly the patient complains of increasing instability.

Treatment

The usual conservative measures are indicated, physiotherapy being particularly important in retaining movement.

Surgery

1 Either arthroscopic or open synovectomy is useful for early disease. It may be performed in conjunction with excision of the radial head
2 In more severe disease, total elbow replacement is the treatment of choice. This would be expected to restore stability and provide a functional range of elbow movement.

Chapter 18

The shoulder and upper arm

Movements of the shoulder are shared between the shoulder joint proper, i.e. between the humerus and glenoid part of the scapula, and movement of the scapula on the chest wall.

Normally, during abduction there is a smooth integration between these movements, but in pathological conditions, one may predominate over the other, e.g. stiffness at the shoulder joint may mean that the only possibility for abduction is at the scapulothoracic joint. On the other hand, stiffness or ankylosis of the sternoclavicular joint may virtually eliminate scapular movements.

The rotator cuff muscles surrounding the upper end of the humerus and the capsule of the shoulder are important for stabilizing the shoulder and producing rotation, while the deltoid provides most of the power of abduction.

Examination

1 Inspection. The patient should be observed standing or sitting in a comfortable position and the levels of the shoulders noted, together with the presence or absence of swellings or wasting. Deltoid wasting accompanies many shoulder conditions, as does wasting of the posterior scapular muscles (supra- and infra-spinatus).

Lecture Notes: Orthopaedics and Fractures, 4e.
By T Duckworth and CM Blundell. Published 2010 by Blackwell Publishing.

2 Palpation. The landmarks are the tip of the acromion, the sternoclavicular joint, the coracoid process and the spine of the scapula. The greater tuberosity of the humerus is also normally palpable. Tenderness is commonly found over the trapezius area, and in capsulitis may be localized to the greater tuberosity. Increase in temperature and boggy swelling may accompany infective conditions or rheumatoid arthritis.

3 Movements. Abduction, flexion, internal and external rotation should be tested (Fig. 18.1). Abduction should be observed from behind to distinguish the various components of this movement. External rotation is tested with the elbow pressed into the side of the body. A useful rapid test is to ask the patient to put his/her hand behind his/her neck and behind his/her back. The patient may avoid attempting external rotation when the joint is unstable, e.g. in recurrent dislocation. The shoulder can sometimes be 'telescoped' upwards and downwards, usually following a paralytic condition such as a stroke.

4 Measurement. The girth of the upper arm may be an index of deltoid or biceps and triceps wasting.

5 Neurology. Damage to the axillary nerve may produce a patch of anaesthesia over the belly of the deltoid. Other shoulder conditions may be associated with brachial plexus injury. Many shoulder conditions cause pain indistinguishable from that due to cervical pathology, so a full neurological examination of the arm is always indicated.

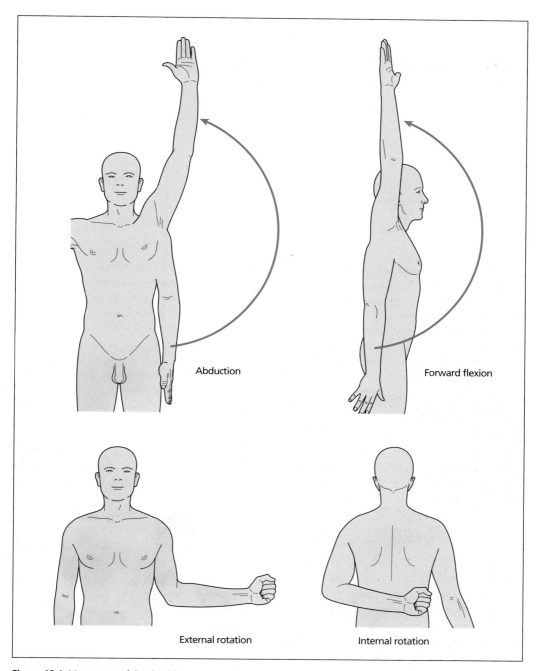

Figure 18.1 Movements of the shoulder.

6 Circulation. The blood supply in the arm may be impaired in certain shoulder conditions which cause pressure on the axilla. Axillary vein thrombosis is an uncommon condition, usually affecting young men and causing swelling and discoloration of the whole arm.

7 Lymphatics. The lymphatic glands in the axilla or supraclavicular fossa may be enlarged from shoulder disease, particularly infective conditions.

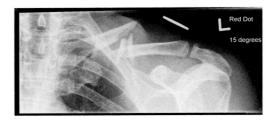

Figure 18.2 Fracture of the clavicle—typical displacement.

Congenital conditions

Sprengel's shoulder

This is a condition in which the scapula is higher and smaller than usual and also rotated into adduction. There may be a ligamentous and bony bar connecting the upper medial border to the cervical spine—the omovertebral bar. This is occasionally worth resecting to give some improvement in appearance: the condition is often associated with Klippel–Feil syndrome (see p. 64).

Developmental conditions

Rarely, recurrent dislocation of the shoulder is due to a developmental defect of the glenoid or humeral head. Constitutional laxity is also an occasional cause.

Traumatic conditions

Fracture of the clavicle

This is one of the commonest fractures in childhood and early adult life, and is usually caused by a fall onto the shoulder or the outstretched hand. The fracture is rarely open. In a child the fracture is usually of the greenstick type.

Clinical features

The patient complains of pain in the shoulder region and supports the weight of the arm with his/her other hand. The bone typically breaks in the middle of the clavicle or at the junction of the middle and outer third. The outer fragment is pulled downwards and forwards by the weight of the arm (Fig. 18.2).

Complications

These are rare, but the brachial plexus may be injured, as may the subclavian artery or vein. Occasionally the dome of the pleura may be penetrated by a bony fragment, producing a pneumothorax. Non-union is very rare and is more likely after internal fixation.

Treatment

For most clavicular fractures, adequate treatment consists of supporting the weight of the arm in a broadarm sling. With the more severely displaced fractures, an attempt is sometimes made to secure a partial reduction by means of a figure-of-eight bandage (Fig. 18.3), but this is not an effective device and may be uncomfortable. Occasionally, displacement may be sufficiently severe to warrant internal fixation, particularly if the fracture is at the lateral end. A small plate or tension band wiring may be used. It should be emphasized that the majority of clavicular fractures heal well, give excellent function and after remodelling are cosmetically satisfactory.

Three weeks of support is normally sufficient and subsequent recovery of function is usually rapid.

Fractures of the acromion and scapula

These are often caused by a direct blow or fall and are rarely displaced. They are usually of little significance. Fractures of the scapula may be associated with rib fractures.

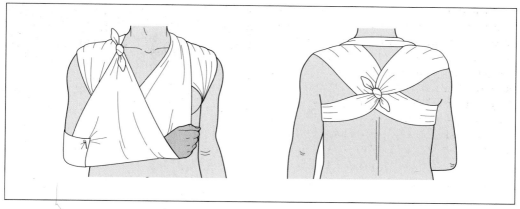

Figure 18.3 Sling and figure-of-eight bandage.

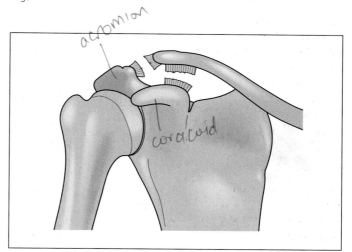

acromion

coracoid

Figure 18.4 Acromioclavicular dislocation.

Treatment

Simple support in a broad sling is sufficient, with early movement when the pain allows.

Subluxation and dislocation of the acromioclavicular joint

These injuries are not common. They are usually caused by a fall onto the shoulder, often as a result of sport. Subluxations of the joint are associated with tearing of the superior and inferior acromio-clavicular ligaments but with the coracoclavicular ligament remaining intact. A complete dislocation also involves rupture of the superior and inferior acromioclavicular ligaments, but in addition the coracoclavicular ligament is also ruptured (Fig. 18.4). In both cases the displacement is difficult to reposition, but function is usually good even without full correction.

Clinical features

The outer end of the clavicle is abnormally prominent and tender, usually with some additional swelling. Shoulder movements are restricted. The injury is frequently missed on X-rays, but the displacement may be more obvious if the patient holds a weight in the hand.

Treatment

A broad sling is often sufficient, sometimes supplemented by strapping over the acromioclavicular joint. The subluxation will usually persist, but function is likely to be normal. Rarely, if pain persists, surgical repair or reconstruction of the coracoclavicular ligament is indicated. The repair may be protected by driving a screw across the clavicle and into the coracoid process, or a threaded pin or figure-of-eight wire may be passed across the acromioclavicular joint. Subluxation may recur when these devices are removed, but the long-term appearance may be improved.

Dislocation of the shoulder

This is a common injury, usually following a fall on the arm or shoulder. It usually occurs in an anterior direction (sub-coracoid) (Fig. 18.5), or occasionally posteriorly or inferiorly.

Clinical features

Diagnosis is usually easy in the typical *anterior dislocation*, because of the flattening of the deltoid muscle, which produces a loss in the curved contour of the shoulder, which therefore becomes 'squared off'. (Fig. 18.6). The injury is painful and the patient

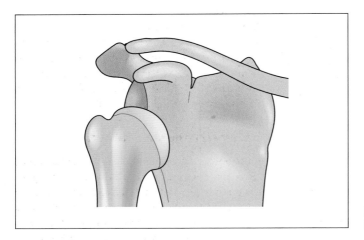

Figure 18.5 Anterior glenohumeral (shoulder) dislocation.

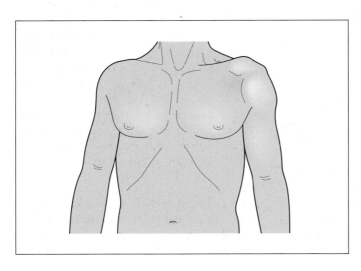

Figure 18.6 Clinical appearance of an anterior dislocation.

supports the arm against all movement. The humeral head may be palpable below the coracoid or in the axilla. *Posterior dislocation* is more difficult to diagnose because the abnormality in contour of the shoulder is less obvious and the X-ray appearances may be misleading, the rotation of the upper end of the humerus producing a so-called 'light-bulb' appearance. The dislocation is best seen on an axillary view if this can be obtained. *Inferior dislocation*, sometimes called 'luxatio erecta', is rare and is characterized by the fact that the arm lies in a vertical position alongside the patient's head. If there is ever doubt about a possible shoulder joint dislocation, a CT scan should be performed.

Complications

Occasionally the circumflex (axillary) nerve is damaged, causing paralysis of the deltoid. This may be checked by testing sensation over the insertion of the deltoid. Recovery is usual. The brachial plexus and axillary artery may also be damaged.

Treatment

Reduction should be carried out as soon as possible. Many methods are available:

1 The patient lies face down with the arm hanging over the side of a couch. With an analgesic injection the muscles gradually relax allowing the operator to slip the humeral head back into the joint.

2 Hippocratic method. The patient is given pain relief and encouraged to relax. With the patient supine, the surgeon pulls downwards on the arm whilst applying counter-traction in the axilla with his/her stockinged foot. This allows reduction of the humeral head into the socket.

3 Kocher's method. The elbow is flexed and traction applied to the arm. The arm is then externally rotated, adducted across the chest and flexed at the shoulder, and then internally rotated until the forearm touches the chest. There is a risk of fracturing the humerus, and the other methods are generally to be preferred.

After reduction an X-ray is taken to confirm the position and the arm is immobilized for 3 weeks in a broad sling. The patient is then encouraged to progressively mobilize the shoulder, often with the help of a physiotherapist. This period is usually shortened in the elderly where stiffness tends to be a problem.

Recurrent dislocation of the shoulder

This occasionally follows one or more traumatic dislocations. It is more frequent if the first shoulder dislocation occurred when the patient was young. After several dislocations a defect may be visible in the head (Hill Sachs lesion) or the edge of the glenoid on a lateral X-ray film (Fig. 18.7), and at operation the cartilaginous glenoid labrum and capsule may be found to be avulsed from the anterior margin of the glenoid (Bankart lesion).

Treatment

Prior to surgical treatment it is important to confirm the direction of dislocation. Operations to stabilize the shoulder are either undertaken as open or arthroscopic (keyhole) procedures. In both situations they involve repairing the damaged capsule and labrum to the glenoid.

Fractures of the humeral neck

These fractures are often classified as abduction or adduction types, depending on the relative positions of the proximal and distal fragments. They are often comminuted, with the greater tuberosity forming a separate fragment. The classification is of little value unless manipulative reduction is to be attempted, in which case it may help to decide if the fracture is stable or unstable. Stable fractures are impacted and may be safely mobilized early. Non-impacted fractures may be considerably displaced and can be associated with damage to the brachial plexus or axillary artery. Many of these fractures occur in elderly people following a fall onto the arm or shoulder. The degree of displacement varies but is often not severe. Despite this, it is unusual for a patient to recover a normal range of shoulder movement following this injury.

Treatment

In this group of patients a broad sling is used to support the arm initially, but mobilization is encouraged as soon as possible. The patient begins to swing the arm in the sling within a few days and

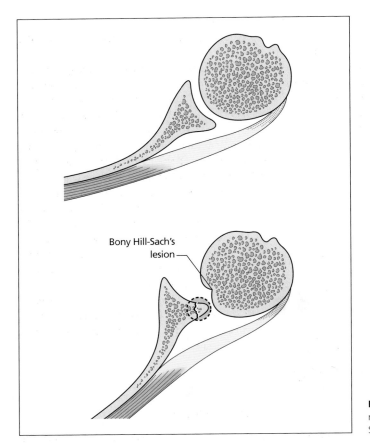

Bony Hill-Sach's
lesion

Figure 18.7 Lateral appearance of a recurrent dislocation showing a Hill Sachs lesion.

as the pain settles more vigorous physiotherapy is commenced.

In younger patients severe displacement may necessitate manipulation under anaesthesia or open reduction and internal fixation. Displacement of the upper humeral epiphysis in a child usually requires manipulation.

Fracture dislocation of the shoulder is a complex injury and priority is usually given to reducing the shoulder dislocation. Severely displaced fractures and fracture dislocations are difficult to manage in all ages and usually require open reduction There may be technical difficulties with open reduction and, even if satisfactory alignment of the fragments is achieved, fixation can present problems. The head of the humerus is not easy to fix adequately. Modern techniques make use of special plates with cancellous screws entering the head (Fig. 18.8). As

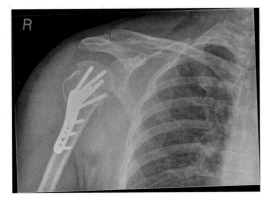

Figure 18.8 Internal fixation of a fracture dislocation of the shoulder.

with the femoral head, ischaemic necrosis of the head of the humerus may occur. In this case, or if it proves impossible to achieve primary fixation, it may be appropriate to replace the humeral head with a prosthesis. This procedure tends to give disappointing results in terms of movements, but may give a reasonably pain-free shoulder.

Fractures of the greater tuberosity may cause a large fragment to be pulled upwards by the rotator-cuff muscles and this may need open reduction and internal fixation to avoid impingement on the acromion.

Fracture of the humeral shaft

This is fairly common in all age groups and may be caused by a fall on the outstretched hand or, more usually, by a direct blow to the upper arm.

Clinical features

There is usually marked swelling and bruising of the arm due to bleeding from the bone and soft tissues. Radiographs often reveal a spiral fracture with displacement making the diagnosis easy.

Complications

The radial nerve is vulnerable as it winds round the shaft of the humerus and is occasionally injured. Rupture of the brachial artery is a rare complication.

Treatment

In principle, this consists of using the weight of the arm to re-align the fragments (Fig. 18.9). A collar and cuff sling, together with gutter-splints surrounding the fracture, extending higher on the lateral side and bandaged in position, is usually adequate. The splints need adjustment weekly in the early stages. As an alternative, a polythene encircling splint fastened by Velcro strips (humeral brace) can be used and the patient can tighten this daily. Immobilization is usually needed for 8–12 weeks. Non-union is relatively uncommon.

Patients who need to be nursed in bed for other injuries or whose fractures fail to align may require internal fixation of the fracture with a plate or intramedullary nail. There are reports of a higher non-union rate with nails and so a return to plate fixation is current practice.

For most purposes with non-operative treatment perfect reduction is not necessary and provided alignment is good, function and appearance will be satisfactory.

Infection

Acute infections

The upper end of the humerus is an occasional site for the development of osteomyelitis. Shoulder movements are usually restricted. Pus may collect under the deltoid or in the axilla. Suppurative

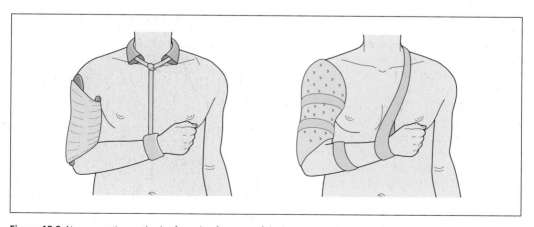

Figure 18.9 Non-operative methods of treating fractures of the humeral shaft.

arthritis of the shoulder is rare and usually occurs in babies or as a complication of rheumatoid arthritis. The sternoclavicular joint is also occasionally the site of acute pyogenic arthritis.

Chronic infections

Tuberculosis may affect the shoulder. It is usually accompanied by severe muscle wasting and stiffness of the joint.

Neoplastic conditions

Secondary neoplasms are not uncommon in the upper end of the humerus, especially from breast carcinoma. Primary neoplasms are rare, but osteosarcoma and osteoblastoma may occur at this site.

Degenerative conditions

The shoulder joint is not commonly affected by primary osteoarthritis but may become degenerate as the result of injury. The joint is not weight-bearing and symptoms are rarely severe enough to warrant surgery. In patients with severe symptoms of pain and shoulder stiffness, shoulder replacement or occasionally arthrodesis of the glenohumeral joint may be considered.

Capsulitis

This is a very common condition. The shoulder is prone to stiffness following a period of immobilization in a sling or following a minor injury. In the majority of patients the symptoms will settle in time. If however the symptoms are interfering with the patient's work or social life, a manipulation of the shoulder under general anaesthesia or arthroscopic capsular release is indicated.

Biceps rupture

Rupture of the long head of biceps from its insertion to the glenoid tubercle is the commonest biceps injury. This results in the 'Popeye' appearance. The patients should be advised that such an injury does not require any treatment. Less commonly the distal biceps may pull from its attachments to the radial tubercle. In this situation the biceps belly appears higher up the arm than on the uninjured side. When this injury is suspected, an ultrasound should be performed to confirm the injury. Surgical treatment is required in this situation with re-attachment of the biceps to the radius.

Inflammatory conditions

Rheumatoid arthritis may affect the glenohumeral joint, the acromioclavicular or occasionally the sternoclavicular joint. In each situation it is important to make sure that the patient is under the care of a rheumatologist and that his/her medical care has been optimized. If symptoms severely affect the acromioclavicular joint, excision of the joint may be extremely helpful. If the glenohumeral joint is chiefly affected, then consideration should be given to joint replacement. This should be expected to reduce the patient's pain, although it is unlikely that normal movement would be achieved. The average range of flexion and abduction after a shoulder replacement is 90 degrees.

Chapter 19

The spine

The vertebral column has a number of different functions.

Stability, support and movement

The spine consists of seven cervical, 12 thoracic and five lumbar vertebra with sacrum and coccyx (Fig. 19.1). Each vertebra is composed of a vertebral body, pedicles, laminae, transverse processes and a spinous process (Fig. 19.2). Intervertebral discs lie between each cervical, thoracic and lumbar vertebra with movement anteriorly occurring at the disc and posteriorly at the two facet joints (synovial joints). Two vertebrae and the disc between form a 'motion segment' (Fig. 19.3). These motion segments allow differing amounts of flexion/extension, lateral bending and rotation with the total movement being considerable. In the thoracic region movement is limited by the ribs and sternum.

The normal spine is straight when viewed from behind but is curved when viewed from the side with the cervical and lumbar spine being lordotic (curve convex anteriorly) and the thoracic spine being kyphotic (convex posteriorly). These normal sagittal curves assist in maintaining balance, but

Lecture Notes: Orthopaedics and Fractures, 4e.
By T Duckworth and CM Blundell. Published 2010 by Blackwell Publishing.

this is largely achieved by large longitudinal, paraspinal muscles running bilaterally up the whole length of the spine and strong ligaments.

Haemopoietic function

The marrow of the vertebral bodies retains its blood-forming capacity throughout life, and vertebrae are, therefore, subject to blood-borne diseases and diseases of the haemopoietic system, such as infection and primary haematological malignancies, e.g. myeloma and metastatic disease. Being cancellous bone, they unite readily after fracturing. Ossification occurs from a single centre in the body and a 'ring' epiphysis for each end-plate.

Spinal cord and nerve root transmission

The spinal cord contains upper motor neurones (UMNs), which are highly susceptible to damage, particularly from rapid compression, movement or ischaemia (failure of blood supply). Once damaged, these UMNs often do not recover even if the cause of the damage is reversed (e.g. compression is removed). There is good evidence that after fracture, decompression makes no difference to the likelihood of neurological recovery. This is thought to be because the damage is done at the time of the injury when the fracture fragments in the spinal

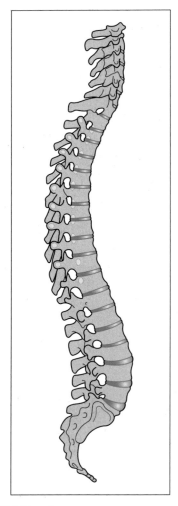

Figure 19.1 The spine.

canal are more displaced than their final resting position.

In slower forms of spinal cord compression, such as metastatic tumour deposits and particularly infection, decompression of the spinal cord can result in improved neurological function. The spinal cord finishes at approximately L1 spinal level in the adult and below this is the cauda equina, which finishes at S2. The nerves within the cauda equina are all lower motor neurones (LMNs) and are less easily damaged by movement or compression, and when there is a motor or sensory

deficit, decompression may produce recovery. The only exceptions are the sacral nerve roots supplying the bladder, bowel and sexual function. If these nerves are compressed, rapid decompression is needed to improve the probability of recovery (cauda equina syndrome). In the spinal cord region, nerve roots exit at every level (LMNs) and these behave in the same way as lumbar nerve roots within the cauda equine, i.e. if there is dysfunction due to compression, decompression may regain function.

History

Most diagnoses can be made from a good history and examination. When spinal pain is the dominant symptom, it is important to decide whether there are any 'red flags'. These suggest more sinister spinal pathology, such as tumour, infection or fracture, and justify urgent referral to an orthopaedic spinal surgeon. If there is any suggestion of early spinal cord compression, emergency referral is needed:

Red flags (see also Box 19.1)

1 New onset of back pain if aged under 10 or over 60 years.
2 Previous history of carcinoma (even if many years ago for breast carcinoma).
3 History of osteoporosis or prolonged steroid use and minor trauma.
4 History of HIV or immunosuppression.
5 Back pain with new systemic sinister features which may themselves need investigation, e.g. unexplained appetite and weight loss.
6 Non-mechanical low back pain, especially with significant night pain and thoracic pain.
7 Rapid onset lower limb neurological symptoms suggesting spinal cord or cauda equina compression.
8 Bladder and bowel dysfunction.

Often patients will present with axial pain (pain related to the axial skeleton, i.e. neck or low back pain) and radicular pain (upper or lower limb pain in a dermatomal or myotomal distribution sugges-

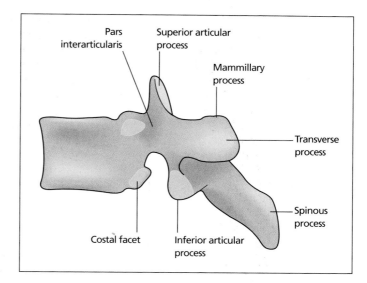

Figure 19.2 Typical thoracic vertebra.

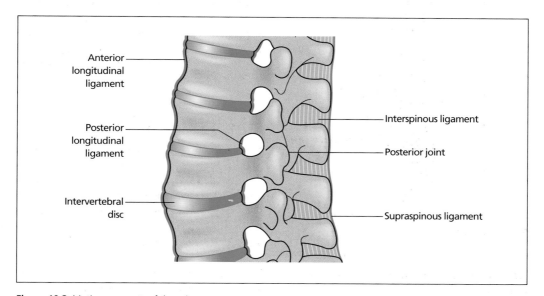

Figure 19.3 Motion segments of the spine.

Box 19.1 Red flag symptoms or history.

- New pain aged <10 or >60
- History of cancer
- Immunosuppressed
- Night pain or thoracic pain
- Rapid onset of neurological symptoms
- Bladder or bowel disturbance

tive of nerve root compression in the cervical or lumbar spine). It is important to determine whether one symptom is dominant or whether the disability is equally from the axial pain and from the radicular pain. This helps guide treatment, as generally, axial pain is difficult to treat with poor success rates whilst radicular pain is easier to treat with higher success rates.

Examination

1 Inspection. The patient should be adequately exposed and viewed standing (or sitting) and the posture of the spine, its shape and any exaggerated or abnormal curves noted. When the patient is viewed from the side, is the kyphosis and lordosis within normal limits and is the patient's trunk angled excessively forwards or backwards? When viewed from the back are there any lateral spinal curves? These are often accompanied by a muscular/rib prominence on the side of the curve, which becomes more pronounced on forward bending (scoliosis) (Fig. 19.4). Is the head positioned above the pelvis or is there any frontal plane imbalance? It is always important to look for skin lesions, such as malignant melanoma, as the trunk is a common site and on the back they can often go unnoticed. A dermatomal rash suggestive of herpes zoster may be the cause of the pain.

2 Palpation. Running the fingers down the spinous processes will detect a localized kyphus or a gap in the ligaments (only present in trauma) and any lateral deviation in the spinous processes will suggest a scoliosis. Occasionally, a 'step' in the spine may help to diagnose a subluxation or spondylolisthesis. Tenderness in the para-spinal muscles is usually only of relevance after trauma. Lipomata are common on the back but if they are close to the midline they need careful evaluation with imaging before any attempted removal as they can communicate with the dural sac.

Temperature differences are rarely felt in spinal disease.

3 Movements. All movements should be tested. Limitation of movement may occur in one direction and not in others. Rotational movements are particularly prone to restriction. Low back pain on forward flexion may suggest the disc as the pain source whilst pain on extension may suggest the facet joints.

4 Measurement is rarely of value in the diagnosis of spinal conditions, except that overall height may diminish progressively in certain diseases, notably osteoporosis. Radiological measurement of the curve size (Cobb angle) is valuable in scoliosis (Fig. 19.5).

5 Neurology. Full neurological assessment of arms and legs is essential in examining any spinal condition. Thoracic lesions may cause girdle pains and anaesthesia around the trunk.

Lasegue's test is performed in patients with lower limb radicular pain (sciatica). The painful leg is passively lifted with the knee extended and when the patient complains of tightness in the back or leg this angle is noted. The angle is then reduced until the tightness just settles and the ankle is dorsiflexed. If the patient experiences his/her usual leg symptoms in the usual distribution, this is then recorded as 'positive tension signs' and it is this finding rather than the reduced straight leg raise that suggests a positive test.

A sensory examination of each dermatome both for light touch and pin prick should be performed, as well as a myotomal examination of muscle strength (L2 = hip flexors, L3 = quadriceps,

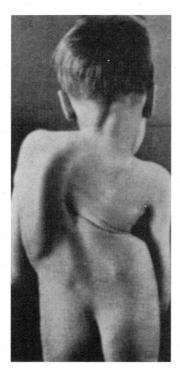

Figure 19.4 Idiopathic scoliosis.

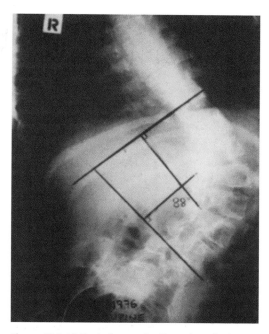

Figure 19.5 Method of measuring X-rays in scoliosis.

L4 = ankle dorsiflexion, L5 = extensor hallucis longus, S1 = ankle plantarflexion).

Upper motor neurone signs, known as long tract signs, suggest pathology within the central nervous system, i.e. brain or spinal cord. These include increased muscle tone (spasticity), brisk reflexes, extensor Babinski reflex and ankle clonus. Long tract signs should always be taken seriously.

6 Circulatory disturbances may be relevant, particularly in a patient with leg pain on walking. This may be due to arterial disease, particularly if the patient is a smoker or diabetic, or may be due to lumbar spinal stenosis. Peripheral pulses must be checked.

7 Lymphatic glands should be palpated, e.g. an acute torticollis may arise secondarily to inflamed neck glands and neoplastic conditions affecting the spine may cause enlargement of glands, e.g. lymphoma.

8 A full general examination, particularly of the abdomen, breasts and urinary system, is always indicated, e.g. an aortic aneurysm may be a cause of chronic back pain.

Traumatic conditions

Stability

In terms of stability, the spine can be considered as an anterior and posterior complex. The anterior complex consists of the vertebral bodies and intervertebral discs, with the posterior longitudinal ligament being its posterior border. The posterior complex consists of pedicles, laminae, facet joints, spinous processes, paravertebral muscles, inter- and supra-spinous ligaments. An injury to one complex is usually stable whilst a two-complex injury is usually unstable and requires surgical treatment (Fig. 19.6). The anterior complex injury is almost always a vertebral body fracture and can be seen on plain radiographs as an anterior wedging of the vertebral body. CT scans are excellent at looking for bony injury and will define the extent of the bony injury, i.e. vertebral body (including any retropulsed fragment back towards the spinal cord or cauda equina) and determine any bony injury to the posterior complex. If the CT scan shows a two-complex injury, it is unstable and usually requires surgical stabilization. If the CT scan shows the bony posterior complex is intact, a significant posterior ligamentous injury needs to be excluded. On clinical examination there may be posterior tenderness, a step or gap between the spinous processes or bruising or swelling. If the clinical examination is normal, in the commonest case of a thoracolumbar fracture, the patient can be gradually sat up and a sitting lateral radiograph performed. If on comparison of the supine and sitting lateral radiographs there is an increase in the kyphosis (anterior wedging at the fracture), this suggests a posterior ligamentous injury and stabilization is required. If there is no increase in kyphosis, the posterior ligamentous complex is intact and the patient can be mobilized and treated conservatively. There is no evidence that brace treatment improves the final result.

Stabilization of the spine is most commonly achieved posteriorly by placing pedicle screws in the vertebra above and below the level of injury and connecting them with a rod on each side to bridge the unstable level (Fig. 19.7).

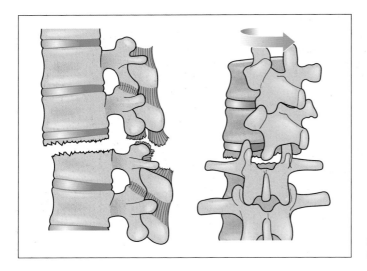

Figure 19.6 Thoracolumbar fracture dislocation.

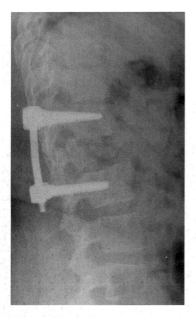

Figure 19.7 Spinal fixation for fracture.

Neurology

A vertebral column injury may or may not result in neurological deficit. Neurological deficit implies the injury is unstable and is likely to require stabilization. Deteriorating neurological function following an injury is an absolute indication for stabilization and possibly decompression. The neurological deficit may be a spinal cord injury (UMN) or may be a cauda equina or nerve root injury.

Spinal cord injury

Fracture is the usual cause with the spinal cord injury occurring at the time of the fracture. The spinal cord injury may be complete or incomplete, although for the first 24–48 hours the spinal cord goes into 'spinal shock' and an apparently complete injury may occasionally be incomplete. Complete motor loss associated with a positive bulbo-spongiosus reflex is a bad prognostic sign. Initial management involves:

1 Avoiding further spinal cord injury by in-line spinal immobilization, log-rolling and rigid cervical collar. The spinal board should be removed on arrival in hospital as this rapidly causes pressure sores

2 Maintaining blood pressure (systolic 90–100 mmHg) and oxygenation to optimize the oxygenated blood reaching the injured cord

3 Urinary catheter (patient will be in urinary retention)

4 Nasogastric tube (for paralytic ileus)

5 Pressure area care.

Patients with complete spinal cord injuries make no recovery and the level of their injury determines function. Thoracic spine injuries result in paraplegia (loss of function and sensation in the lower limbs, including bladder and bowel control). Cervical spine injuries result in paralysis with a varying degree of upper limb involvement depending on the level (quadriplegia). Complete spinal cord injuries above C4 seldom survive as diaphragmatic function is lost and there is no voluntary respiratory function.

Patients with incomplete spinal cord injuries always make some recovery. It is rarely a complete recovery but they will usually walk. At the initial neurological examination, patients with incomplete spinal cord injury may just have a flicker of movement in the big toe or perianal sensation, so a careful and complete neurological examination is essential.

Other causes of spinal cord injury are tumour and infection (see below).

Cervical spine

These injuries must always be considered as the consequences of a missed injury may be a permanent spinal cord injury. They should always be suspected in unconscious patients, patients with significant trauma (high-speed road traffic accident, falls from a height) and particularly in patients reporting even very mild neurological symptoms following an accident. For example, a patient with tingling in the distribution of an upper limb nerve root may have a cervical unifacet fracture or dislocation (Fig. 19.8). The thoracic and lumbar spine should be assessed clinically and a complete neurological examination of upper and lower limbs performed.

A lateral radiograph of the cervical spine is the first investigation and the C7/T1 junction must be visible for the radiograph to be considered adequate (Fig. 19.9). This radiograph should be inspected for:
1 Adequacy
2 Bony alignment
3 Vertebral body fractures
4 Facet joint fractures/dislocations
5 Spinous process fractures

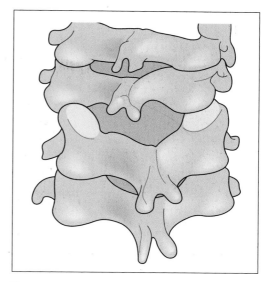

Figure 19.8 Cervical subluxation.

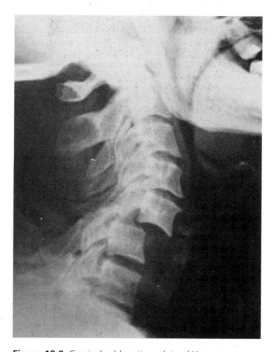

Figure 19.9 Cervical subluxation—lateral X-ray.

6 Increased soft-tissue shadow anteriorly suggestive of injury

An AP and open mouth view should also be obtained.

The indications for a CT scan of the cervical spine are:

1 Fracture visible or suspected on radiographs
2 Neurological deficit
3 Head injury requiring CT scan.

An MRI scan should be performed if there is any neurological deficit and in cervical facet dislocations before reduction as a significant disc protrusion within the spinal canal may cause a neurological deficit on attempted reduction of the dislocation.

In the unconscious patient, it is generally accepted that the cervical spine can be cleared if a consultant radiologist finds no evidence of bony injury on a cervical spine CT scan. The hard collar can be removed, making nursing much easier and reducing the risk of an occipital pressure sore. When the patient becomes alert enough for a clinical examination of the neck, this should be performed. A normal CT scan does not exclude an unstable cervical spine due to disc disruption at the front and a ligamentous injury at the back, i.e. no bony injury, but fortunately these are extremely rare.

If a cervical spine fracture is diagnosed or if the patient is unconscious, the thoracic and lumbar spine should be imaged using either plain radiographs or CT scans with sagittal (lateral) reconstructions.

Treatment depends on the degree of instability with more stable injuries being treated with a rigid collar (Aspen or Philadelphia, see Fig. 24.9, p. 230); slightly less stable injuries in a halo-vest (a halo is fixed to the skull using four diagonally placed screws and the halo is then connected by lateral posts to a lined non-removable polyethylene jacket); and unstable injuries being treated by anterior and/or posterior instrumented stabilization and fusion with the aim being to fuse as few motion segments as possible.

Fractures of the atlas (C1, Jefferson fracture)

The ring of the atlas is usually fractured in four places as a result of a vertical compression force. This is usually a stable injury and spinal cord damage is uncommon. They are difficult to detect on plain radiographs but diagnosis is confirmed on CT. Treatment in a collar is usually adequate.

Fractures of the odontoid peg (C2)

These are common and easily missed. The fracture is usually at the base of the peg and displacement may be considerable, while still allowing survival. A lateral radiograph often shows the fracture with the degree of angulation and displacement. In young patients, treatment is either halo-vest immobilization for 8–12 weeks or stabilization with anterior screws across the fracture (only certain fracture patterns are suitable). Non-union is reported in 30–70% and is treated with a C1/2 posterior fusion. Elderly patients do not tolerate a halo-vest and are treated in a rigid collar. Non-union (pseudarthrosis) usually occurs in the elderly but is fairly stable and does not cause symptoms.

Hangman's fracture (C2/3 traumatic spondylolisthesis)

Pedicle fractures of C2 allow forward subluxation of C2 on C3. There are degrees of severity of this injury and traction is rarely needed. When required, however, it should only be applied by a spinal surgeon familiar with these injuries as severe distraction and spinal cord injury can occur in some types of this injury. The less severe forms of this injury can be treated with a rigid collar or halo-vest immobilization, whilst the more severe form requires anterior C2/3 discectomy and fusion (iliac crest bone graft + anterior plate).

Subaxial injuries (C3–C7)

Vertebral body fractures can be relatively stable, requiring only collar immobilization, or may be completely shattered with posterior complex injury requiring corpectomy (removal of the fractured bone) and reconstruction with iliac crest bone graft and an anterior plate with or without posterior stabilization. In more severe injuries, spinal cord injuries are common.

Facet joint dislocations may be unilateral or bilateral and may be associated with fracture of the facet joint. They are usually detected on the lateral radiograph by anterior subluxation of the superior vertebral body on the inferior vertebral body. A 25% subluxation suggests a unifacet problem, whilst a 50% subluxation suggests a bifacet dislocation (Fig. 19.9). Early reduction is advised, ideally after an

MRI scan to exclude a large protrusion within the spinal canal. Reduction is best performed using skull traction and by gradually increasing the weight with the neck flexed. With each additional 10 lb, a clinical examination and lateral radiograph should be performed. Weights should be increased to a maximum of approximately 40% body weight. Once the reduction is achieved, the neck is extended and most of the weights removed. These injuries, even when reduced, are often unstable and require anterior (or posterior) stabilization.

Isolated spinous process injuries are stable and require only symptomatic treatment.

Whiplash injuries

These are usually considered to be soft-tissue injuries to the neck or low back from motor vehicle accidents, usually when the patient's car is hit from behind. The symptoms are usually of pain in the neck, sometimes with radiation down the arm and occasionally with paraesthesiae or numbness in the arm or hand. The onset of symptoms is often delayed by a few hours or even days. The neck is usually stiff and there may be objective neurological signs. Radiographs are usually normal or show degenerative changes only and treatment is conservative with analgesia and early mobilization. The prognosis is variable; most patients recover completely, others continue to have troublesome symptoms over a long period and occasionally the disability proves to be permanent.

Thoracic spine

In thoracic spine fractures it is important to determine whether the sternum has been fractured, as this makes instability and progressive kyphotic deformity much more likely.

Osteoporotic wedge fractures

Minor trauma, even sneezing, may cause anterior thoracic wedge fractures in patients with known osteoporosis, or they may be a first presentation of osteoporosis. Analgesia and possibly brace treatment (for comfort) along with treatment of the osteoporosis is sufficient for most fractures with the pain gradually settling. If the pain fails to settle

after 3–6 months, vertebroplasty or kyphoplasty can be performed. This involves inserting a hollow probe down the pedicle of the collapsed vertebra, from posteriorly using image intensifier (X-ray) guidance. Bone cement is then injected. Pain is usually significantly improved but risks include cement leakage around the spinal cord with paralysis and adjacent level vertebral fractures.

Fracture dislocations

These usually occur after high-speed road traffic accidents with the injury usually in the upper to mid-thoracic spine. Complete neurological deficit is common. These fractures require stabilization because if left untreated the deformity is often painful and fixation is thought to reduce the risk of an ascending syrinx (cyst within the spinal cord), which may result in upper limb neurological problems if the syrinx ascends into the upper thoracic and lower cervical spinal cord.

Thoracolumbar spine

Fractures at the thoracolumbar junction are the most common spinal fracture and their management is considered above.

Lumbar spine

These can be considered in the same way as thoracolumbar fractures, but are usually stable and seldom require surgery. If the patient presents with cauda equina syndrome due to a fracture fragment compressing the cauda equine, then this should be decompressed urgently to increase the probability of return of bladder and bowel function. Nerve root injury may recover with conservative treatment, but decompression should be considered if there is bony compression or significant disability from leg weakness or pain. Decompression should always be accompanied by stabilization with pedicle screws and rods.

Sacrum and coccyx

Sacral fractures occur from direct impact or are associated with pelvic fractures. They may produce neurological problems, particularly affecting the bladder, and often cause long-term pain. 'Sacral insufficiency' fractures occur in patients with osteoporosis, with the pain usually settling to a tolerable level.

Coccydynia is a condition in which there is chronic pain in the coccygeal region, often following an injury or after childbirth, but sometimes for no obvious reason. The pain is much worse on sitting. It is difficult to cure, but may be helped by injections of local anaesthetic and steroids with manipulation of the coccyx via the rectum under general anaesthesia. Excision of the coccyx may be necessary, but is not always curative.

Infection

Infection of the spine involves the disc space with destruction of the disc and the vertebral body end-plates. Infections are usually pyogenic with *Staphylococcus aureus* being the most common (especially in children) followed by Gram-negative organisms. Tuberculosis is again becoming increasingly common and should always be considered. Patients will usually present with constant, severe and worsening back pain, which can be in any region. Neurological symptoms are uncommon but can occur as a result of an epidural abscess or from vertebral body collapse with spinal cord or cauda equina compression over the apex of the resulting kyphosis (see Fig. 13.4). The diagnosis should always be suspected in anyone who is immunocompromised and who presents with new-onset back pain, i.e. HIV, steroid users, diabetics, chemotherapy.

It is essential that an organism is obtained *before* commencing antibiotics. Investigations should include a full blood count, where there is usually a raised white cell count, and inflammatory markers (ESR and CRP) are usually very elevated. Blood cultures are positive in 50%. An MRI scan confirms the diagnosis. A biopsy can be guided using CT or plain radiographs (image intensifier). Once an organism has been obtained, antibiotics are started intravenously and continued for 10–14 days, and if the patient is responding symptomatically and the inflammatory markers are reducing, they can be

changed to oral antibiotics to complete a 3-month course. For some reason, *Staph. aureus* infections usually result in a spontaneous anterior fusion and symptoms settle. If pain persists, a spinal stabilization and fusion with instrumentation may be necessary.

Degenerative conditions

Degenerative spinal disease is most common in the cervical and lumbar spine, and the same principles apply to both regions.

Low back and neck pain

Low back and neck pain can be caused by arthritis of the synovial facet joints, disc degeneration, muscular pain and ligamentous pain, and may be multifactorial as well as affecting multiple levels of the spine. Unfortunately, there is no accurate and reproducible feature of the history or examination, and no specific investigation to decide which structure and at which level the pain is originating from. For this reason the management of low back and neck pain is generally conservative, involving analgesics, physiotherapy and general advice to stay active and help to realise that pain does not indicate damage to the spine.

However, it is vital that serious spinal pathology is excluded and for this reason 'red flags of serious spinal pathology' have been developed (Box 19.1, p. 159). Non-spinal causes for low back pain should also be considered:

1 Abdominal aortic aneurysm
2 Pancreatitis
3 Urinary tract infection/pyelonephritis.

Surgery for neck pain alone is generally not beneficial, although cervical disc replacements may have a role when pain can be reliably identified as coming from a single level.

In the lumbar spine, spinal fusion is the 'gold standard' treatment for low back pain in suitable patients who fail conservative treatment for at least 6 months. Suitable patients are those with one or two degenerative intervertebral discs on MRI scan (although this is found in 20–40% of the population who do not suffer from low back pain).

Spinal fusion involves permanent immobilization of the presumed painful spinal segment and can be done from the front of the spine, from the back of the spine or both. Results show approximately 50% of patients achieve a significant (not total) improvement in their symptoms. More recently, lumbar disc replacements have been shown to be as effective as spinal fusion.

Radicular pain

Upper and lower limb pain may be due to pain referred from structures in the neck or low back, e.g. painful facet joints. This is known as referred pain and treatment is directed at the neck or low back. Limb pain may also come from a nerve root(s) and this is known as radicular pain. Radicular pain tends to follow a dermatomal distribution, usually has a sensory abnormality and may produce motor weakness. In the lower limb this is referred to as sciatica. Pain which passes below the elbow or knee is usually radicular whilst pain confined to the proximal segment is often referred. However, C5 radicular pain does not extend below the elbow and this is common; and L2 and L3 radicular pain does not extend beyond the knee and this is relatively common.

Disc protrusion

In young patients (<40 years), a disc protrusion is the commonest cause of radicular pain and in the lumbar spine it usually occurs at L4/5, compressing the L5 nerve root, or L5/S1, compressing the S1 nerve root. Straight leg raise on the affected side is reduced with positive tension signs (exacerbation of leg symptoms on dorsiflexing the ankle). Sensory testing may reveal an abnormality and for L5, extensor hallucis longus (big toe dorsiflexion) may be weak and for S1 tip-toe stance may be weak. S1 radicular pain often results in an absent ankle reflex.

Radicular pain is often severe but 85% of cases settle in 2–3 months. Sufficient, regular analgesia should be prescribed with advice to avoid prolonged bed rest. Patients should be referred to a spinal surgeon if symptoms are too severe to be controlled with oral analgesia or are not resolving after 6–8 weeks. If MRI confirms the diagnosis, a lumbar micro-discectomy will significantly improve the leg pain in 90% of patients. Patients usually only spend one night in hospital and are back at work in 4–6 weeks (8 weeks for manual labourers). Radicular pain in the upper limb is usually treated with anterior cervical discectomy and fusion, again with excellent results.

Cauda equina syndrome

It is essential to ask about bladder and bowel dysfunction with typical symptoms being urinary incontinence in women, urinary frequency or urgency and altered perianal and genital sensation. Any abnormality should result in a careful digital rectal examination, which should include pinprick sensation around the perianal margin and an assessment of anal tone and squeeze. This examination should be carefully documented and abnormality should prompt emergency referral to a spinal surgeon. These symptoms and signs are important because compression of the cauda equina (usually by a central disc protrusion) compresses the sacral nerve roots supplying the bladder and bowel and sexual function. These nerves are particularly sensitive to compression and should be decompressed as soon as possible to give the best chance of recovery.

All patients with sciatica should be warned about the symptoms of cauda equina syndrome and advised to seek urgent medical attention if they develop.

Facet joint degeneration

In older patients radicular pain may be due to a disc protrusion but is more commonly due to facet joint hypertrophy compressing the nerve root (or the uncovertebral joints in the cervical spine). In these patients straight leg raising is usually full with negative tension signs. Sensory, motor and reflex abnormalities may be present, as seen in younger patients with disc protrusions.

The differential diagnosis should include:

1 Peripheral vascular disease (check peripheral pulses)
2 Hip or knee osteoarthritis
3 Diabetic or other neuropathy
4 Polymyalgia rheumatica
5 Motor neurone disease
6 Multiple sclerosis.

As for disc protrusions, 85% of episodes of radicular pain settle within 2–3 months. Patients should be referred to a spinal surgeon if symptoms are too severe to control with oral analgesia or are not resolving after 6–8 weeks. An MRI scan will confirm the clinical findings and a microscopic nerve root decompression will significantly improve leg pain in 85% of patients. Again, the equivalent procedure in the neck is an anterior cervical discectomy and fusion, with excellent results.

Central stenosis

Spinal cord

'Stenosis' means narrowing and the clinical consequences of narrowing of the central spinal canal depend on the site and speed of the compression.

Slow compression in the spinal cord region is due to degenerative changes and results in cervical or thoracic myelopathy. Early symptoms of cervical myelopathy include clumsy hands (inability to do fine motor tasks and poor handwriting), ataxia (poor balance whilst walking), altered lower limb sensation (often bilateral) and bladder and/or bowel dysfunction. Early upper motor neurone signs are imbalance on eye closing (Romberg's test), increased muscle tone, hyper-reflexia, ankle clonus and extensor plantar responses. Thoracic myelopathy is similar but without the upper limb symptoms.

Subacute compression, i.e. rapidly progressive symptoms, is usually caused by tumour or infection and failure to detect the early symptoms or signs will result in sensory and motor deficit, which following a decompression will sometimes recover but often does not. Therefore early diagnosis is essential.

Sudden, rapid compression of the spinal cord is usually caused by trauma and results in complete or incomplete spinal cord injury (see above).

Cauda equina

Slow compression of the cauda equina results in lumbar spinal stenosis, which presents with leg pain on walking or prolonged standing. The pain is usually in the buttock, back of the thigh and calf, and may be accompanied by radicular pain if the degenerative process has also caused nerve root compression. Patients will usually describe a diminished walking distance and the pain will settle if they stop and either sit down or bend forward as flexion of the lumbar spine increases the cross-sectional area of the lumbar spinal canal. Symptoms usually take a few minutes to settle, unlike the situation in peripheral vascular disease where leg pain from ischaemic claudication settles in approximately 30 seconds. The patient's partner will often comment on how the patient bends forward when walking and to this end, the patient may even use a stick. Motor weakness may occur if nerve roots are involved, but bladder and bowel dysfunction is very rare as the degenerative change resulting in facet joint hypertrophy is a very slow process and the nerves seem to accommodate to this slow compression.

Examination should include an assessment of peripheral pulses. An MRI scan will show which levels are affected; with the L4/5 level being the most common.

Not all patients have progressive symptoms and a lumbar epidural injection of steroids and physiotherapy may be all that is required. The surgical treatment traditionally involves decompression of the lumbar spine (removal of the ligamentum flavum and laminae centrally and partial excision of the facet joints to free up the involved nerve roots). This is a very successful operation with 75% of patients achieving good to excellent results. A newer treatment involves placing a device (metal or plastic) between the spinous processes, resulting in interspinous process distraction at the involved level, and this distraction and localized flexion of the spine results in an increase in the cross-sectional area of the spinal canal. Long-term results are not available.

Subacute compression results in lower limb sensory disturbance, motor weakness and bladder and bowel dysfunction. There are no upper motor neurone signs as compression is below the spinal cord. Reflexes may be absent. Causes include tumour, infection and kyphotic spinal deformity. Sensory and motor deficits respond well to decompression but bladder and bowel dysfunction needs to be treated as an emergency, as for rapid onset cauda equina syndrome.

Rapid compression of the cauda equina results in cauda equina syndrome (see above) and although usually caused by a disc protrusion, may be caused by tumour, infection, trauma and haematoma.

Neoplastic conditions

Almost all malignant tumours of the vertebral column are metastases with common primary sites including breast, lung, prostate, kidney and gastrointestinal system. Patients may present with a history of a known malignancy which may go back many years, especially in malignant melanoma and breast carcinoma, or this may be the first presentation. Other common malignancies include myeloma and lymphoma. Back pain and/or neurological compromise are the usual symptoms with examination findings depending on whether the central compression involves the spinal cord or cauda equina. If there is no known primary site, a careful history and examination should be performed, including breast and prostate examination. Appropriate blood tests should be requested, including tumour markers. A CT scan of the chest and abdomen is needed, looking for the primary site (lung or kidney) and other secondary deposits in the lung or liver. In cases where there is an unknown primary, excluding renal carcinoma is essential as surgery on renal metastases can result in fatal haemorrhage unless pre-operative embolization is performed. An MRI scan of the whole spine will reveal all metastases and confirm the level of spinal cord/cauda equina compression.

In patients with back pain but no neurological deficit, it may be appropriate to treat the metastasis with radiotherapy if the primary site is known, but this will depend on the responsiveness of the metastasis to this treatment. If the metastasis is known to be unresponsive to this treatment, surgi-

cal stabilization with instrumentation may be needed. In patients with partial neurological deficit, a decompression and stabilization (with pedicle screws and rods) is required. It is essential that the patient's symptoms are detected early and any upper motor neurone symptoms or signs (see above) must be taken seriously, as neurological deficit from spinal cord compression will often not recover following decompression and ideally the patient should be diagnosed before onset of neurological symptoms or at worst when they are only mild.

Deformity

The commonest type of spinal deformity is scoliosis, which is a lateral curvature of the spine associated with rotation. This usually affects teenagers, with larger curves being eight times more common in girls than boys. There is no known causation, although genetic factors are known to be important and abnormalities of neuro-central control are likely mechanisms. This type of scoliosis is therefore called adolescent idiopathic scoliosis (see Fig. 19.4) and the curve progresses during the adolescent growth spurt. The commonest curve site is in the thoracic spine, resulting in a rib prominence to the side of the curve and causing significant cosmetic deformity in these teenage girls (Fig. 19.10). Brace treatment is of unproven benefit, although it is still offered in many centres. Surgery is for cosmetic reasons and for larger curves which are known to progress after skeletal maturity. Surgery involves either anterior or posterior partial correction of the deformity using instrumentation. The aim is to use the instrumentation to hold the spine in the corrected position whilst the spine fuses. In general, in adolescent idiopathic scoliosis, curves greater than 50 degrees will continue to progress slowly once skeletal maturity is reached, but will only cause cardiorespiratory morbidity if a thoracic curve reaches 90 degrees. Otherwise patients are more likely to develop back pain and surgery does not seem to improve this.

Other causes of scoliosis include:
1 Infantile and juvenile idiopathic scoliosis. This is also of unknown cause and treatment is

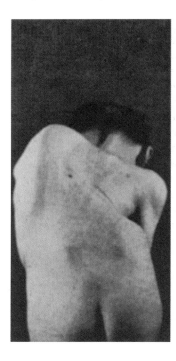
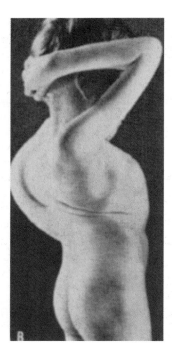

Figure 19.10 Idiopathic scoliosis showing rib hump.

similar to that for adolescent idiopathic scoliosis, but with some treatments trying to maintain spinal growth in these very young patients. Infantile idiopathic scoliosis may require plaster-cast and brace treatment

2 Neuromuscular causes. Duchene muscular dystrophy, other myopathies, Friedreich's ataxia, spinal muscular atrophy and cerebral palsy are all common causes of scoliosis, and often require surgery for progressive deformity and sitting imbalance, as these patients are often in a wheelchair.

3 Syndromic. Many syndromes are associated with scoliosis.

4 Congenital scoliosis. Hemi-vertebrae (wedge-shaped vertebrae) are the commonest problem and these produce either scoliosis, kyphosis or a combination of the two depending on the orientation of the hemi-vertebra. These often cause curve progression, especially if combined with an abnormal fusion of the vertebrae in the concavity of the curve (concave bar). Treatment involves either a non-instrumented fusion on the convex side or excision of the hemi-vertebra.

Metabolic conditions (see Chapter 14)

Osteoporosis is the most common form of metabolic bone disease affecting the spine and can result in vertebral body fractures, often following only minor trauma. Treating patients who have sustained a vertebral osteoporotic fracture with bisphosphonates (which inhibit osteoclast bone resorption) and calcium supplements reduces the risk of further osteoporotic fractures at all sites.

Other metabolic spinal conditions include Paget's disease (increased bone turnover with poorly formed new bone), where pathological fractures and spinal stenosis can occur, and osteomalacia (a bone mineralization problem secondary to vitamin D deficiency), which produces pain, proximal muscle weakness and sometimes vertebral body fracture.

Rheumatological conditions (see Chapter 10)

The management of these patients is largely medical.

Rheumatoid arthritis tends to involve the C1/2 region with instability common and surgical stabilization sometimes required. Newer disease-modifying treatments may reduce the incidence of these problems.

Ankylosing spondylitis results in bony ankylosis (fusion) of the spine, including the sacroiliac joints (see Fig. 10.4). This often results in a kyphotic deformity of the whole spine, which can make it impossible for the patient to look straight ahead and may require one or more spinal osteotomies to correct the deformity. A completely rigid spine is also more susceptible to fracture. If a fracture occurs and the spine is deformed it is essential that the patient is not forced into a 'normal' anatomical position on a spinal board or cervical collar as this position is not 'normal' for that patient and may result in spinal cord injury.

Other seronegative arthropathies such as psoriatic arthropathy, Reiter's syndrome and enteropathic arthropathy, can all produce spinal pain which tends to be inflammatory and is improved by non-steroidal anti-inflammatory medication.

Chapter 20

The pelvis

Examination

The examination of the pelvis forms part of the examination of both the lumbar spine and the hip and is dealt with in Chapters 19 and 21.

Traumatic conditions

Fractures of the pelvis

Pelvic fractures are common, particularly following road and industrial accidents. The associated soft-tissue injuries are usually more serious than the fractures themselves.

Stable fractures

The true pelvis forms a ring structure which is intrinsically stable. Fractures which do not enter the ring or which break it in one place only are stable, e.g. fractures of the iliac wing or pubic bones (Fig. 20.1a–c). They may be associated with bleeding, but other complications are rare.

Treatment
This consists of rest until the patient can walk, usually after 2–3 weeks.

Lecture Notes: Orthopaedics and Fractures, 4e.
By T Duckworth and CM Blundell. Published 2010 by Blackwell Publishing.

Unstable fractures

These are fractures in which the pelvic ring is disrupted in two or more places, one of which is above the level of the hip, e.g. through the waist of the ilium, the sacroiliac joint or sacrum. Various combinations are possible (Fig. 20.1e–g). Many of these injuries are produced by compression forces, either from front to back or from side to side, as may occur if the patient is crushed by machinery or run over by a vehicle. A double fracture below the level of the hip joints is technically unstable, but may be treated as stable (Fig. 20.1d).

Displacement

The pelvis may open like a book or one side may be displaced upwards—hindquarter dislocation. Either of these is likely to be associated with bladder or urethral damage. Occasionally, if the fracture is produced by side-to-side compression, the fragments of the pelvic ring may overlap, narrowing the ring. In addition to standard AP X-ray films, inlet and outlet views and CT scanning of the pelvis may be necessary to make an accurate diagnosis.

Treatment
The management of the fractures themselves is usually relatively simple, but that of the complications is much more difficult. The unstable open book-type fracture will often close if the patient is turned on one side. Some form of fixation is required and the current trend is to use a specially

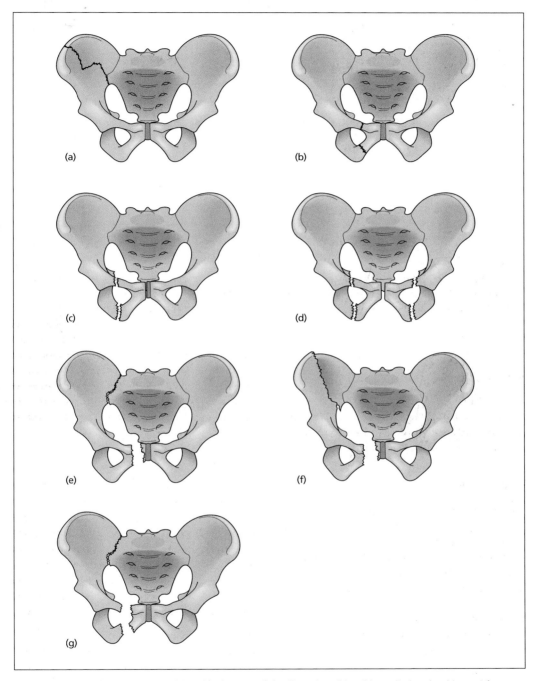

Figure 20.1 Fractures of the pelvis. (a) Stable fracture of the iliac wing; (b) stable undisplaced pubic rami fractures; (c) stable, displaced fractures of the pubic rami; (d) stable saddle fracture of pubic rami bilaterally; (e, f, g) unstable vertical shear fractures of the right hemipelvis.

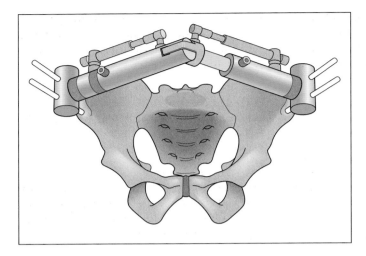

Figure 20.2 Fixation with external frame.

designed external frame with bone screws introduced at various points around the iliac crest (Fig. 20.2). This technique, if properly applied, gives firm fixation. It may then be possible to mobilize the patient, although standing and walking is not usually advised for the first few weeks. An alternative method to treat open book-type injuries is internal fixation of the symphysis.

Vertical unstable fractures cannot be controlled definitively by external fixation and traction. Referral to a specialist centre for treatment is required. There these fractures are often stabilized both anteriorly with a plate and posteriorly with screws across the sacroiliac joint.

The unstable fracture usually requires 12 weeks of fixation before stability is achieved. If the sacroiliac joint has been damaged by the fracture, the patient may later complain of chronic pain in this area and fusion of the joint may become necessary. Distortion of the true pelvis does not usually cause symptoms unless the hemi-pelvis height is disturbed. This can result in leg length or seating balance disturbance. Interference with childbirth is uncommon.

Complications

Haemorrhage
All pelvic fractures produce some bleeding, but this can be catastrophic from the large plexus of vessels which line the inside of the pelvis. Internal bleed-

ing can be recognized by the usual signs of impending shock and by the palpation of a mass in the suprapubic region and particularly on rectal examination. Pelvic bleeding is one of the causes of shock which should be considered in the patient with multiple injuries, and an X-ray of the pelvis is regarded as routine in such patients. If there is a palpable suprapubic mass an ultrasound must be carried out and the level should be marked on the abdomen to assess whether it is increasing in size.

Treatment
This involves blood transfusion, sometimes massive, and often, for this reason, requiring fresh blood. Stabilizing the fracture helps to control the bleeding and should be done as soon as possible. If frame fixation is not readily available, a pelvic binder may be used as a temporary measure or for definitive treatment. If control of the bleeding is not achieved, arteriography and selective embolization of leaking arteries is indicated. It may be possible to ligate a major bleeding vessel or, alternatively, the wound may have to be packed if the bleeding is venous and is otherwise not controlled. Control may still not be possible and death can occur from exsanguination.

Injuries to the bladder and urethra
These are common and diagnosis may be difficult. The badly injured patient may not be able to pass

urine for many reasons, such as fear, shock or pain, as well as damage to the bladder or urethra.

The bladder may be ruptured either intra- or extra-peritoneally. The urethra may be ruptured anywhere along its length in the male, but particularly at the junction of the prostatic and membranous parts.

Diagnosis

The patient may be asked to pass urine, but not to persist if the attempt fails. Percussion of the bladder is helpful in that a distended bladder cannot have been ruptured, but urethral injury is still a possibility. Rectal examination may reveal a pelvic swelling representing blood in the pouch of Douglas. With a rupture of the membranous urethra, the prostate may be displaced upwards and be impalpable. There may be bleeding from the urethra.

Investigations and treatment

There are at least two schools of thought.
1 A soft catheter is passed gently down the urethra. If this passes easily into the bladder and a moderate quantity of clear or slightly blood-stained urine is obtained, the system is usually intact and the catheter is left *in situ*. If the catheter fails to pass, this may be because the urethra is damaged. In this case there is often bleeding *per urethram* and bruising in the perineum. Urethroscopy may be helpful in making the diagnosis. If the catheter passes into the bladder and blood or a very small quantity of urine is obtained, the bladder may be ruptured and a cystogram is advisable. In either of these cases, surgical exploration will be necessary.
2 Catheterization is considered dangerous and suprapubic drainage is established if the patient fails to pass urine. The bladder or urethral rupture is then investigated at leisure and repaired as appropriate.

Injuries to the rectum

These are less common. They may be suspected by the presence of bleeding *per rectum* and diagnosed by rectal examination and sigmoidoscopy. They are usually treated by suture and a temporary colostomy with thorough washout of the bowel distal to the perforation.

Vaginal injuries

These are also uncommon. They are treated by suture.

Sciatic nerve injuries

These are relatively uncommon. Recovery may occur, but occasionally the nerve is trapped in the fracture and persistent pain may result. Exploration may be necessary to free it.

Neoplastic conditions

The upper end of the femur and the pelvis are common sites for the development of metastatic carcinoma. Pathological fracture of the pelvis is uncommon. Radiotherapy is used to control the local tumour, and fractures frequently unite.

Primary tumours are much less common, but osteosarcoma, osteoclastoma and chondrosarcoma are all seen in this area. Radical resection is sometimes feasible with replacement with a prosthesis or allograft.

Metabolic disorders

Demineralizing conditions may result in collapse or deformity of the hip joint with stress fractures in the femoral neck. This is particularly noticeable in those conditions arising during growth, i.e. rickets and renal osteodystrophy where the femoral neck may be grossly abnormal with slipping of the epiphysis. In osteomalacia, 'Looser's zones' may be seen in the rami of the pubis and ischium and occasionally in the femoral neck.

Paget's disease commonly affects the pelvis and upper end of the femur (see Chapter 14).

Chapter 21

The hip and thigh

Development of the hip joint

The femoral head and acetabulum develop in early embryonic life as a unit. Acetabular development depends on the head of the femur being in its normal position, and on movement of the joint. If the femoral head is out of place, the acetabulum develops poorly. A second 'false' acetabulum may indeed develop higher up in the iliac bone itself. The femoral neck is anteverted relative to the shaft of the femur, and the angle of anteversion gradually diminishes after birth. The acetabulum on the other hand usually points backwards (retroverted) to a variable degree to match the anteversion of the femoral neck. In untreated developmental dislocation of the hip (DDH, see below), the neck usually remains anteverted with the acetabular orientation being abnormal. The epiphysis of the femoral head normally develops at the age of 4–5 months. Stability of the hip depends upon the shape of the joint, the capsule and ligaments, and the control exerted by the muscles around the hip.

Examination

1 Inspection. At the start of any hip examination the patient should be asked to walk. Various types

Lecture Notes: Orthopaedics and Fractures, 4e.
By T Duckworth and CM Blundell. Published 2010 by Blackwell Publishing.

of gait may be apparent. If the hip is painful, an 'antalgic' gait may occur, with the patient spending as little time as possible on the painful hip. A flexion deformity of the hip may reveal itself by the patient tilting the pelvis forwards and arching the lumbar spine to bring the trunk upright (Fig. 21.1).

Another common gait often seen in abnormalities of the hip is the 'Trendelenburg' gait. As the patient walks, the pelvis tilts down on the opposite side of the diseased hip. The reason for this abnormal gait is that the abductor muscles (gluteus medius and gluteus minimus) do not work properly in the presence of hip disease (Fig. 21.2). Such a gait is seen in conditions such as:

1 Dislocation of the hip (especially DDH). The stable pivot of the hip joint in the acetabulum is lost

2 A painful hip joint, as in osteoarthritis. The Trendelenburg gait sometimes seen in osteoarthritis probably relates to painful inhibition of the action of the gluteal muscles

3 An abnormality of the femoral neck, either being short or in a varus position.

The patient should then be examined lying down. Abnormal rotation of the leg is common with femoral neck fractures. Typically, the leg is shortened and externally rotated on the side of a femoral neck fracture. The leg may also be short but not particularly rotated in significant osteoarthritis of the hip, where loss of the femoral head contour leads to shortening of the limb.

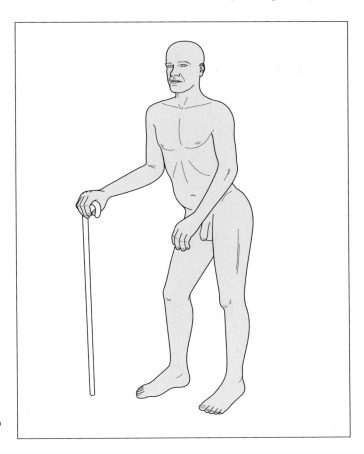

Figure 21.1 Stooped posture due to flexion contracture of the hip.

Evidence of muscle wasting, scars and sinuses related to deep infection around the hip should be looked for.

2 Palpation. The bony landmarks around the hip are the anterior superior iliac spine, the greater trochanter, the ischial tuberosity and the pubic symphysis. Tenderness is difficult to elicit in hip disease, as the joint is deep seated. Tenderness over the greater trochanter is not indicative of hip joint pathology itself, and may be due to trochanteric bursitis (see below).

3 Movements. The hip joint has a wide range of movements. These are classified as:

  1 Flexion and extension

  2 Abduction and adduction

  3 Internal and external rotation.

Flexion of the hip is important for normal gait, and particularly stair climbing, getting in and out of chairs and the bath. Flexion of the normal hip is usually limited by impingement of the thigh on the lower abdomen. Extension of the hip is less important, and may be less than 10–15 degrees. Fixed flexion of the hip joint may develop in osteoarthritis, and is elicited using the 'Thomas's test' (Fig. 21.3). This is an important test to understand. Fixed flexion in the hip is demonstrated by flexing the opposite hip as far as it will go. This effectively flattens any lordosis of the lumbar spine, and reveals any fixed flexion deformity on the examined side. Abduction and adduction are tested by moving the joint whilst the examiner keeps a hand on the opposite anterior superior iliac spine to detect pelvic movement. Normal range is from 40 to 50 degrees of adduction to 40–50 degrees of abduction.

Internal and external rotation of the hip can be assessed with the hip in extension, by rolling the

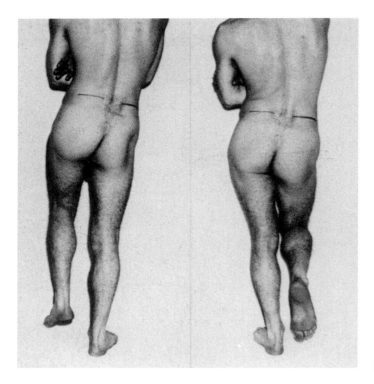

Figure 21.2 Trendelenburg test.

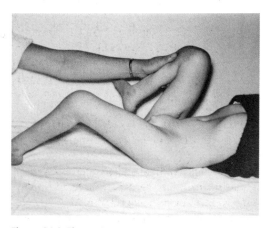

Figure 21.3 Thomas's test.

tive to the spine, such shortening can be masked when the patient stands up. The 'apparent length' of the limb is therefore measured from a mid-line point (e.g. xiphisternum) to the medial malleolus. If such a pelvic tilt occurs, then real and apparent lengths may be different (Fig. 21.4). Even though the 'shortening' is only apparent, the patient will still notice that the leg feels short.

Paediatric hip conditions

A child with hip disease may not present with pain or a history of trauma but with an unexplained limp. Unexplained knee pain should raise the suspicion of hip abnormality.

leg in and out on the bed, using the foot as a pointer. Rotation in flexion is also assessed, with the hip at 90 degrees of flexion.

4 Measurement. The 'true length' of the limb can be measured from the anterior superior iliac spine to the medial malleolus. If the pelvis is tilted rela-

Developmental dysplasia of the hip

(See Chapter 8, p. 52.) Newborn babies are screened for the possibility of DDH by careful examination of the knee in the neonatal period. Most at risk are those babies born to families with a positive family

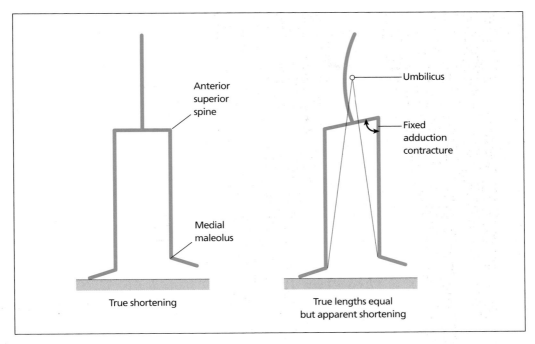

Figure 21.4 True and apparent leg shortening.

history, or with breech presentation. Ultrasound scanning should detect most at-risk cases, but late presentation may occur as delay in walking, a limp or a leg length discrepancy. Missed DDH often leads to a non-congruent joint and the early development of osteoarthritis in adult life.

Perthes disease

This is a condition seen most commonly in boys between the ages of 5 and 10. It is considered to be due to segmental avascular necrosis of the femoral head with associated disintegration, and subsequent healing and deformity. A limp, hip pain or knee pain may be the presenting feature. The clinical signs are usually minor, perhaps slight restriction of movements of the hip, especially internal rotation, associated with some spasm.

X-rays

1 The earliest sign is increased density of the epiphysis and widening of the medial joint space. The changes may occupy all or part of the head (Fig. 21.5), and a lateral film is helpful in judging prognosis.

2 Later, the epiphysis appears fragmented and the head may show signs of flattening (Fig. 21.6). The overlying articular cartilage survives and the head may be more normal in shape than the X-ray suggests. The metaphysis may be widened and show cystic changes.

3 Healing occurs with gradual re-absorption of the dense bone and laying down of normal-looking new bone.

4 Restoration of the bone occurs over the course of several months. The head may be left flattened, widened and with a wider neck (Fig. 21.7).

5 Remodelling may occur until growth ceases. There is evidence that the risk of developing osteoarthritis in later life is proportional to the distortion of the head at the end of the growth period.

Treatment

There is much argument about treatment and some authorities only treat the child until the

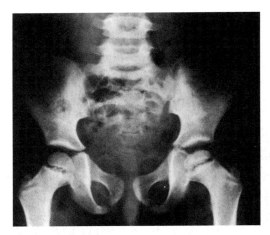

Figure 21.5 Perthes disease—early stage with increased density of the epiphysis.

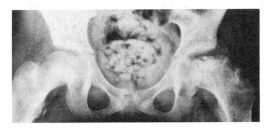

Figure 21.6 Perthes disease—showing fragmentation of the head.

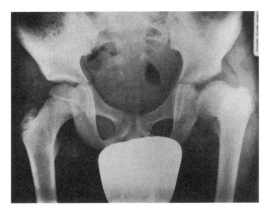

Figure 21.7 Perthes disease—at the end of the period of regeneration.

immediate symptoms settle—usually over 2–3 weeks. A short period on traction will usually achieve this. Others believe that distortion of the head can be prevented by various measures: conservative and surgical. Many regimes are practised, but none of them has been fully evaluated because of the difficulty of making clinical comparisons. There is a gradually developing agreement that putting the hip in internal rotation and abduction may help to contain the epiphysis within the acetabulum and prevent distortion whilst it is still in the plastic stage.

Conservative

The position of abduction and internal rotation may be achieved either by traction in bed or on an abduction frame, or without traction, in abduction plasters or an abduction brace. Treatment may be provided in hospital or at home, and some of the regimes allow sufficient mobility to enable the child to attend school.

The value of non-weight-bearing is uncertain; some allow full weight-bearing in plaster cylinders, others insist on strict bed rest. Some surgeons abduct and internally rotate the hip, then bring the leg down to neutral by carrying out an osteotomy through the intertrochanteric region. They claim this shortens the period of immobilization and achieves equally satisfactory results.

Prognosis

The prognosis is better in the younger child and when only part of the head is involved. Girls fare worse than boys for any given age. Many of the difficulties centre around treating a condition which quickly becomes symptom-free and is then only manifest as a series of changes on X-rays.

Slipped upper femoral epiphysis

This is a condition whereby the developing epiphysis of the hip, often in an overweight hypogonadal boy, partially slips, leading to hip pain or referred pain to the knee. Diagnosis may be difficult and therefore delayed, but a 'frog lateral' X-ray will show the deformity (Fig. 21.8). The condition requires urgent surgical stabilization with

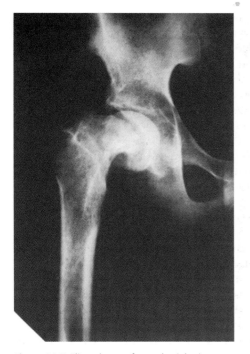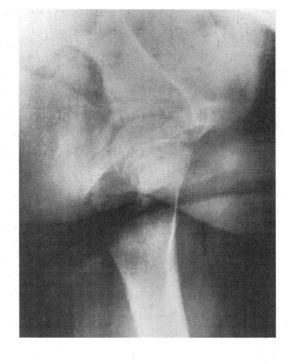

Figure 21.8 Slipped upper femoral epiphysis.

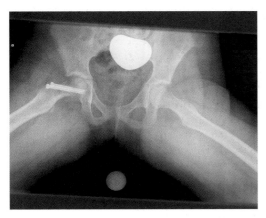

Figure 21.9 Internal fixation of a slipped femoral epiphysis.

pins to prevent further slippage of the epiphysis (Fig. 21.9). The contralateral hip is at high risk of slippage, and patients and parents should be warned to return if any further knee or hip pain occurs.

Septic arthritis

Septic arthritis is occasionally seen in children. The diagnosis should be suspected if a child presents who is ill, toxic and unable to walk. The child will often be extremely irritable, and movement of the affected joint will not be possible because of pain. Diagnosis is confirmed by a raised white cell count and erythrocyte sedimentation rate. Urgent surgical drainage is important to reduce the risk of late degenerative change developing. *Staphylococcus aureus* is the usual infective organism.

Irritable hip or transient synovitis

An effusion may occur in the hip of children in association with a generalized viral illness. These children are not unwell and can move the hip, although there is a degree of stiffness present. Ultrasound scanning may demonstrate an effusion, and the condition usually resolves spontaneously.

Adult conditions

Pain from the hip joint is usually felt in the groin, or on the lateral or anterior aspect of the thigh. It is very common for hip pain to be referred to the knee, and the hip should always be examined if a patient presents with knee pain. Buttock pain is less commonly associated with the hip joint itself, and is usually caused by lumbar spine disease. Disorders of the hip often affect walking distance, produce a limp, and lead to stiffness, which affects the patient's ability to perform activities of daily living. A flexible hip is required to negotiate steps, stairs, to put on shoes and socks, and to get in and out of the bath.

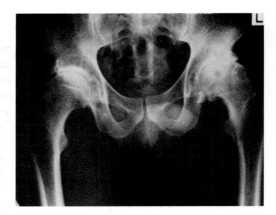

Figure 21.10 X-ray appearance of osteoarthritis of the hip.

Osteoarthritis

The hip is one of the joints most commonly affected by osteoarthritis. In the majority of cases there is no obvious reason for the development of the degenerative changes. In some cases there may be a relevant history of hip disease, such as DDH, Perthes disease or other childhood problems. There may be a history of previous trauma to the hip or pelvis, or other arthritic processes leading to hip joint destruction (e.g. rheumatoid arthritis). The peak incidence of hip arthritis is in the sixth decade. Bilateral hip disease is often seen.

The predominant symptoms of osteoarthritis of the hip are pain felt in the groin or anterior thigh. The pain is made worse by walking, and can keep the patient awake at night when the arthritis is well advanced.

The typical signs of osteoarthritis of the hip include a limp, an antalgic or Trendelenburg gait. Flexion and adduction deformity are commonly seen, leading to shortening of the limb. The Thomas test may reveal a fixed flexion deformity (see Fig. 21.3).

The X-ray signs of osteoarthritis of the hip include joint space narrowing, subarticular cysts, peripheral osteophytes, and subchondral sclerosis (Fig. 21.10).

Treatment

Conservative treatment of hip disease should always be tried first. Patients should be encouraged to lose weight, use a stick to offload the hip joint itself, and use appropriate analgesics or anti-inflammatory medication as necessary.

If these measures are ineffective, then total hip replacement should be considered. Total prosthetic joint replacement in the hip was pioneered in the early 1970s by Sir John Charnley and others, following largely unsuccessful attempts at joint resurfacing using cup arthroplasties or acrylic femoral head replacements. Most designs of hip replacement have a metal femoral stem and an ultra-high-molecular-weight polyethylene ('UHMWPE') acetabular component (Fig. 21.11). Implants can be fixed to the underlying bone with polymethyl methacrylate bone cement or may be 'uncemented'. Various surface finishes have been applied to prosthetic surfaces to encourage bone ingrowth, including beads, mesh and plasma-sprayed titanium. Hydroxyapatite is a synthetic bone substitute, and has been applied to many prostheses to encourage bony incorporation. Alternative bearing surfaces, such as ceramic on ceramic or metal on metal bearings, are becoming more popular, as there is good evidence that particles of UHMWPE are responsible for the loosening process that is observed in hip replacement patients. Each step the patient takes with a metal on UHMWPE bearing may liberate millions of wear particles, which escape into the joint space. These may gain access to the bone cement interface by cracks in the cement mantle, and those particles in

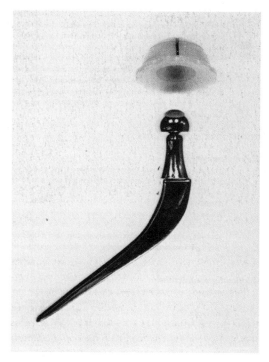

Figure 21.11 Charnley hip prosthesis.

the submicron range (<1 μm in diameter) may be taken up by macrophages. The macrophages are unable to digest the particles and in the process produce cytokines, which activate local osteoclasts, producing unopposed bone loss and ultimately leading to prosthetic loosening.

Over 45 000 total hip replacements are performed in the UK each year. The procedure is now highly developed, and over 90% of patients have an excellent outcome from surgery. Data from the Swedish Hip Registry suggest that patients should expect a greater than 80% chance of their hip replacement lasting more than 20 years.

Risks
The significant risks of the surgery include:
1 Infection. This may occur in approximately 0.5% of patients, and can have significant consequences. The prosthetic joint will require removal to eradicate the infection, and once the infection has settled a further joint may be inserted. Total hip replacement is performed in ultra-clean air theatres, with antibiotic prophylactic cover, by surgeons and assistants usually wearing body exhaust gowns.

2 Thromboembolism. Fatal pulmonary embolism may occur in between 1 in 200 and 1 in 300 patients. Deep vein thrombosis is seen clinically in perhaps 1 in 20 patients after hip replacement, and patients are given thromboembolic prophylaxis to reduce the incidence of deep vein thrombosis. There is little evidence so far that thromboembolic prophylaxis has an effect on the fatal pulmonary embolism rate.

3 Dislocation. The ball and socket of the hip joint may come apart if the patient twists or bends without care. Dislocation may require a manipulation of the hip under anaesthesia. The risk of dislocation is low at between 1% and 2%.

Other arthritides

Rheumatoid arthritis, psoriatic arthritis and ankylosing spondylitis can produce hip disease and associated pain. Total hip replacement is often indicated in these conditions.

Paget's disease

The pelvis is often involved in Paget's disease, and can produce hip pain. Bisphosphonate medication is useful in the treatment of Paget's, but co-existent osteoarthritis of the hip can also occur.

Avascular necrosis

Avascular necrosis (AVN) of the femoral head can lead to an effusion in the hip joint, causing pain and stiffness, but if the process continues the femoral head may collapse, producing secondary osteoarthritis. MRI allows the diagnosis to be made in the early stages, but if radiological evidence of AVN is present, surgical treatment to arrest the disease is less successful. Arthroplasty may be required. The causes of avascular necrosis are:
1 Idiopathic
2 Excess alcohol
3 Sickle cell disease
4 Prolonged steroid therapy

5 Working in pressurized environments (e.g. deep sea divers)

6 Malignancy.

The proximal femur is a common site for metastatic malignancy. Treatment with radiotherapy or bisphosphonates may slow the disease progress. Prophylactic stabilization of impending fractures may be worthwhile if the tumour occupies more than 50% of the diameter of the bone. Primary bone tumours as a cause of hip pain are extremely rare.

Infection

Primary septic arthritis of the hip is very rare in adults, but may be present in immunocompromised patients. The incidence of septic arthritis of the hip in intravenous drug abusers appears to be rising, especially if intravenous injection has been attempted in the groin. Surgical drainage is usually necessary. Ultrasound scanning may be required to demonstrate the presence of an effusion.

Tuberculosis (TB) of the hip is occasionally seen in the UK, especially in immigrants. TB of the hip, however, is much more common in underdeveloped countries. The infection may develop in the metaphysis of the femur and may quickly spread to involve the whole of the hip joint. The joint surfaces are destroyed, and the capsule becomes distended with pus. This may break through to the surface of the skin, forming a sinus, which may become secondarily infected.

The management of TB relies heavily on antibiotic therapy with drainage of chronic abscesses and removal of necrotic bone. Patients with TB treated as children may present in later life for consideration of hip replacement.

Painful soft-tissue conditions around the hip

Trochanteric bursitis is a self-limiting inflammation of the bursa between the greater trochanter and the fascia lata. The condition is characterized by pain over the tip of the greater trochanter, rather than pain in the groin, and usually settles with anti-inflammatory medication or occasionally with a steroid injection.

Fractures

Fractures of the femoral neck

Fractures of the neck of femur (NOF) are epidemic in the developed world, usually secondary to osteoporosis. Femoral neck fractures may occur occasionally in young patients through normal bone, but the energy required for such an injury to occur is usually very high.

In osteoporotic NOF fractures, the bone is by definition pathological, and the injury required to produce the fracture is often minimal. A trivial fall may lead to an NOF fracture, and indeed some patients describe their hips collapsing whilst they are standing, perhaps suggesting that the femoral neck breaks without a fall at all!

The mental and social condition of the patient at the time of injury is all important in determining the ultimate outcome of all femoral neck fractures. Relatively few patients return to full mobility following these injuries. The patients are often elderly and frail, and co-existent medical conditions may need to be assessed and treated prior to surgical treatment of the fractures.

Intracapsular fracture

This type of fracture occurs through the femoral neck just below the head of the femur. A history of a fall is common, and the patient will be unable to weight bear. The hip is very painful to examination, and the leg is held in a short and externally rotated position.

The survival of the patient is the first consideration with this fracture, which carries a poor outcome: 30–40% of patients die within the following 12 months. Early mobilization is essential to avoid the complications of long periods confined to bed. Two methods of surgical treatment are available:

1 Reduction of the fracture and internal fixation. The fracture is reduced on the operating table under X-ray control, and two to three screws are passed across the fracture to stabilize it (Fig. 21.12). This technique is most successful in minimally displaced fractures, where the blood supply to the

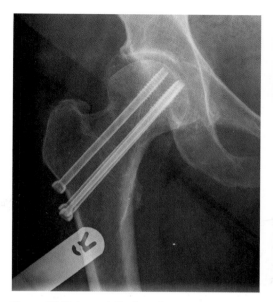

Figure 21.12 Internal fixation of an intracapsular hip fracture.

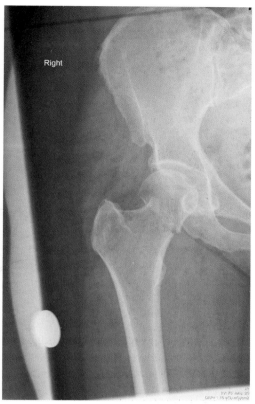

Right

Figure 21.13 Subcapital hip fracture.

head of the femur is unlikely to have been damaged by the fracture.

2 In displaced fractures, the blood vessels on the posterior aspect of the femoral neck may be torn, and the blood supply to the head of the femur may be compromised significantly (Fig. 21.13). In displaced fractures it is preferable to remove the ball of the femur, and replace it with a prosthesis. An Austin Moore or Thompson's implant is often used, to allow early weight-bearing (Fig. 21.14). Total hip replacement may be preferable in younger patients.

Intertrochanteric fractures

These fractures are 'extracapsular' and occur in the wide metaphyseal region between the two trochanters in the femur. Because the blood supply to the fracture is adequate, such fractures tend to unite without difficulty. Patients present in a similar way to those with subcapital fractures, and X-ray diagnosis is usually straightforward (Fig. 21.15).

Internal fixation of intertrochanteric fractures with the 'dynamic hip screw' (DHS) is the preferred treatment method (Fig. 21.16). Such a device

allows controlled collapse of the fracture when the patient is weight-bearing to encourage union of the fracture. As the fracture heals, some shortening may occur.

Fractures of the femoral shaft

These fractures are seen in all age groups. The fracture may occur at various levels in the shaft of the femur, and is frequently an open injury and associated with other injuries. Bleeding at the site of the fracture can often be significant, and blood replacement may be necessary. Injuries to the femoral and sciatic nerve occasionally occur.

The immediate treatment of a femoral shaft fracture is the application of a Thomas splint (see Fig. 5.5, p. 36). This applies counter-traction to the limb, and the resulting stability aids in reducing blood

185

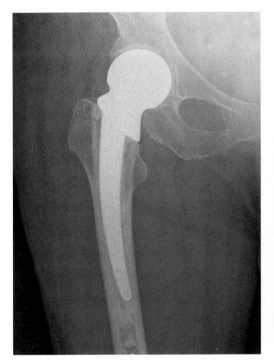

Figure 21.14 Cemented hip hemi-arthroplasty for hip fracture.

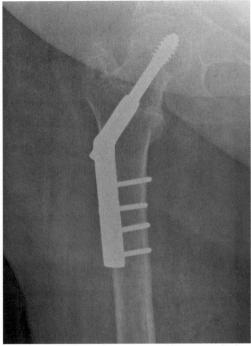

Figure 21.16 Dynamic hip screw used to treat an intertrochanteric hip fracture.

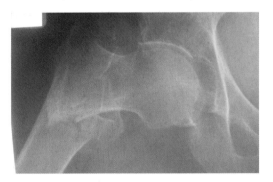

Figure 21.15 Intertrochanteric hip fracture.

loss from the fracture, and in providing comfort for the patient. Gallows traction is a simple method of applying traction in a child aged up to 2 years (see Fig. 5.7, p. 38).

The preferred treatment of femoral shaft fractures is fixation with an intramedullary nail. The intramedullary nail is inserted under X-ray control from the greater trochanter, passed down across

the fracture, and locked both below and above the fracture with cross-screws to stabilize the fracture in rotation. Modern intramedullary nails are often made of titanium, and allow immediate mobilization. Full weight-bearing is usually possible from 3–4 weeks after intramedullary nailing. Union usually occurs by 12–16 weeks from the time of fracture. Knee stiffness is often seen, but usually resolves with exercise. Anterior cruciate ligament rupture is commonly associated with fractures of the femoral shaft.

Fractures of the distal femoral shaft and supracondylar fractures

These fractures are often displaced by the action of the gastrocnemius muscle attachments. The treatment of such fractures is commonly surgical, and a variety of different devices are available. Intramedullary nail fixation is possible, the nail being passed through the knee, across the fracture, and

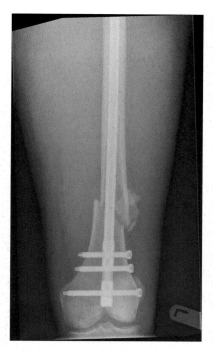

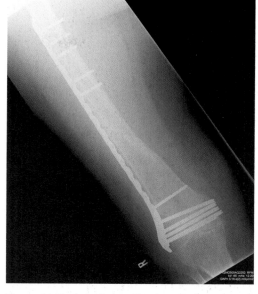

Figure 21.18 Locked plate for distal femoral fracture fixation.

Figure 21.17 Intramedullary nail for femoral fracture.

locked as described above (Fig. 21.17). Intramedullary nail fixation is good provided bone quality is adequate. In the presence of osteoporotic bone, locked plate fixation is now becoming more popular (Fig. 21.18). The comminuted fracture fragments are held together with screws connected to a plate applied to the side of the femur. These plates may be inserted through relatively small incisions and serve to 'bridge' the fracture site.

Dislocations

The hip joint is anatomically strong, but dislocation can occur, usually as a result of considerable violence. These injuries are often caused by car accidents in which a front seat traveller is involved in a head-on collision and strikes his/her knee under the dashboard. Depending on the degree of flexion of the hip, a simple dislocation may occur or there may be a fracture dislocation involving the head or acetabulum. The acetabular fracture may be through the back, the floor or, less commonly, the front of the acetabulum.

Simple dislocation of the hip is usually posterior. It is very rare in children. The patient presents with the leg flexed, adducted and shortened, and the femoral head may be palpable in the buttock. The sciatic nerve, particularly the lateral popliteal division, may be damaged.

Treatment

Reduction is usually easy. It is carried out under general anaesthesia with the patient lying supine, preferably on the floor or a low couch, and by flexing the hip and simply lifting the head of the femur into the joint. Once reduced, it is usually stable and the leg is then held on longitudinal skin traction for 3 weeks to allow the capsule to heal, followed by a further 3 weeks of protected weight-bearing. Stiffness of the joint is rarely a problem.

Chapter 22

The knee and lower leg

Knee conditions present in a wide variety of ways and affect all age groups.

Applied anatomy

The knee is not a simple hinge joint. The femoral condyles are of different lengths and flexion occurs by a mixture of gliding and rolling of the condyles on the tibia. Rotation of the tibia is important at the end of extension as the femur is screwed into medial rotation relative to the tibia, the 'locking-home' mechanism.

The menisci are the 'shock absorbers' of the knee and share the load transmitted across the joint. They are mainly avascular structures and, if torn, healing only occurs if the meniscus is detached from the capsule along its vascular edge. The cruciate and collateral ligaments are normally tight when the knee is extended. In the flexed position, some medial and lateral tilt is possible. The anterior cruciate ligament controls forward movement of the tibia on the femur and the posterior cruciate controls backward movement.

The muscles moving the knee, particularly the quadriceps and hamstrings, contribute considerably to its stability and can compensate for some ligamentous injuries.

Lecture Notes: Orthopaedics and Fractures, 4e.
By T Duckworth and CM Blundell. Published 2010 by Blackwell Publishing.

Examination

1 **Inspection**
- **Gait.** The patient with a painful knee usually walks with the knee held stiffly and quickens the step on the affected side, a so-called antalgic gait. A patient with a fused knee has difficulty swinging the leg through and will circumduct (swing the leg out) or 'vault' (rise up on the standing leg) to stop the foot hitting the ground.
- **Deformity.** Flexion deformities are common. A 'locked' knee is one which will not extend fully. Abduction and adduction deformities are also common—*bow leg* (*genu varum*) and *knock knee* (*genu valgum*). If these deformities are long-standing they predispose to arthritis. Wasting of the quadriceps is almost invariable with knee pathology. It is usually most obvious in the fleshy belly of vastus medialis. Generalized swelling of the knee is usually due to an effusion or to synovial thickening. Cystic degeneration of a meniscus may cause a localized swelling over the joint line and is more common on the lateral side. Other swellings around the knee include the so-called 'Baker's cyst' (posteriorly), a semi-membranosus bursa (postero-medially), and pre-patellar and infra-patellar bursae over the patella and tibial tubercle, respectively.

2 **Palpation.** The useful landmarks are the patella, tibial tubercle, head of the fibula, and the medial and lateral joint lines between the femoral and

tibial condyles. Some practice is needed to locate these accurately. An effusion fills up the hollows on either side of the patella. If the effusion is large, the patella 'floats' off the femoral condyles and it can be tapped backwards against the condyles ('patellar tap'). A small effusion can be detected by stroking the fluid out from one of the hollows into the supra-patellar pouch and back again, watching for the bulge to appear. Synovial thickening has a 'boggy' consistency and the whole synovium is often tender. Localized swellings should be palpated carefully and an attempt made to determine their attachments. Classically, a semi-membranosus bursa disappears in flexion. Tenderness is often well localized, e.g. over the medial or lateral joint line or over one or other attachment of the collateral ligaments. Increased temperature may be felt over an inflamed synovium or over neoplasms or infections around the knee.

3 Movements. Active and passive flexion and extension should be tested. Extension beyond 0 degrees is called 'recurvatum'. It is not uncommon in teenage girls. The normal knee flexes until the calf meets the thigh. The normal range of movement is 0–150 degrees but varies from patient to patient.

4 Special tests. In the knee the special tests are for ligamentous instability and meniscal tears.

To test the *collaterals*, the knee is held in full extension, and then an attempt is made to rock it into varus or valgus. This movement may be painful if it stretches a strained ligament. In the fully extended position, the knee will only 'rock' if one of the collaterals and the posterior cruciate is torn. If the test is repeated with the knee in 15–20 degrees of flexion, the cruciates are relaxed and the knee will 'rock' if a collateral ligament alone is torn.

The *cruciates* are tested by the examiner flexing the knee to 90 degrees (if possible) with the sole of the patient's foot on the couch. He/she then sits on the foot to stabilize the leg and attempts to draw the tibia forwards or push it backwards relative to its neutral position. If the posterior cruciate is torn, the tibia will fall backwards a little and the knee will look slightly flattened when viewed from the side (posterior sag).

Lachmann's test is more sensitive and is only concerned with the *anterior cruciate ligament (ACL)*. The knee flexed 10–15 degrees and an attempt is made to draw the tibia forwards on a fixed femur. The pivot shift attempts to mimic the instability or giving way the patient experiences with ACL deficiency. The leg is held in slight flexion, internal rotation and a valgus axial load is applied whilst extending. The knee will jump if positive. This is a hard test to master.

McMurray's test is for *meniscal tears*. The knee is flexed as far as possible and the compartment to be tested is loaded whilst the knee is rotated, with the operator feeling for a click or clunk. Though this test is widely taught in clinical practice it is rarely used as it has low specificity.

5 Measurement. The girth of the thigh is a useful measure of quadriceps wasting. The two sides should be compared by measuring up from a fixed point (e.g. the joint line) and noting the circumference. Knock knee may be estimated by measuring the distance between the malleoli with the knees touching in full extension.

6 Neurology, vascularity and lymphatic drainage. Sensibility, major pulses and examination for oedema should all be tested for routinely in the examination of the knee.

Congenital and developmental conditions

These are dealt with in Chapter 8.

Trauma

Dislocation of the knee

This is rare but serious and signifies a very severe injury, e.g. a high-speed motorcycle crash. It is associated with rupture of ligaments and the direction of dislocation is variable. It may be associated with other life-threatening injuries and with damage to the popliteal artery and peroneal nerve.

Treatment
The patient is stabilized using ATLS principles and the knee can then be addressed. Initial reduction is

by manipulation and vascular repair if necessary. An MRI scan will determine which ligaments are torn. Modern surgical repair or reconstruction of all ligaments yields better results than simple immobilization.

Dislocation of the patella

This is an injury of children and young adults, usually from a fall or blow to the side of the knee. The patella dislocates laterally and the knee remains flexed until the patella is reduced. The injury involves a tear of the medial capsule and quadriceps expansion. Some knees seem to be prone to recurrent dislocation and patients with this tendency exhibit the so-called 'apprehension sign' if an attempt is made to dislocate the patella laterally.

Treatment

Reduction can usually be achieved by straightening the knee. A short period in a cast or firm bandage to allow the capsule to heal can be followed by active mobilization. Recently, interest has focused on the medial patellofemoral ligament which can either be repaired or reconstructed.

Ligamentous injuries

The cruciate ligaments and the collateral ligaments are frequently injured, especially in sportsmen. Incomplete healing may lead to long-term instability of the joint, with a feeling of 'giving way'.

Strains of the collateral ligaments

These are common following sporting injuries. As the ligaments lie outside the knee joint, the knee has no effusion but pain is present on palpation of the injured structure. Stressing the ligament causes pain, but the joint remains stable. Medial collateral ligament strains are more common than those affecting the lateral ligament.

Treatment

These injuries usually settle with a short period of rest, followed by support and exercises.

Complete ruptures of the collateral ligaments

These are diagnosed by demonstrating clinical instability. When tested by varus or valgus stressing, an isolated collateral ligament rupture will not result in significant instability if the test is performed with the knee fully extended, but at 10 degrees of flexion there will be significant opening of the joint on the damaged side. If significant laxity is present, particular attention should be paid to the anterior and posterior cruciates. An MRI scan is particularly helpful when the knee is painful and difficult to examine.

Anterior cruciate ligament tears

This very important injury is still sadly often missed in the A&E department. Any sportsman or woman who has a history of twisting the knee, who heard a snap or pop and was unable to continue playing due to a swollen painful knee can be assumed to have an ACL tear until proven otherwise. Injuries sustained in sports such as skiing, netball, football and rugby should alert the physician. As the incidence is around 30 per 100 000 population per year, a large district hospital will see approximately 100 new injuries per year. Often the patient has a medial collateral and lateral meniscal injury as well (the so-called 'unhappy triad'). The diagnosis is made from the history, but the presence of an effusion or haemarthrosis and a positive 'draw sign' (Fig. 22.1) also give clues. The 'Lachmann's test' is more sensitive.

Posterior cruciate tears

Posterior cruciate tears are less common, typically occurring in goalkeepers or in dashboard injuries. Other ligament injuries should be suspected, particularly to the so-called posterolateral corner. Posterior instability is diagnosed by the posterior 'sag' with both knees flexed to 90 degrees and by a posterior draw sign.

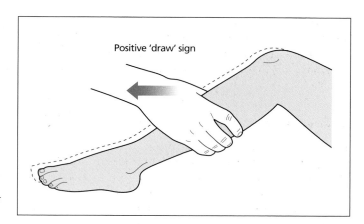

Positive 'draw' sign

Figure 22.1 Diagnosis of an anterior cruciate tear.

Diagnosis and treatment of ligamentous ruptures

In the acute setting, these injuries are very difficult to diagnose accurately due to pain and swelling. They tend to be classified in terms of the direction of instability, e.g. lateral, posteromedial, etc. It may be necessary to carry out a full examination under anaesthesia to assess what type or combination of instability is present.

Repair of isolated cruciate ruptures by simple suture is unlikely to be successful unless the ligament has avulsed a fragment of the tibial spines (usually in young people), in which case this may be fixed back surgically with a more predictable result.

For any injured knee, early movement is advisable, if necessary using a hinged brace. Only if the knee is locked (unable to extend) do patients with acute ACL ruptures require urgent surgery. Normally the knee is allowed to settle with physiotherapy and, later, a decision about reconstructive surgery is made. Younger patients who are active sporting participants are more likely to require early reconstruction. Older patients may have a period of conservative treatment with reconstruction only being advised if the knee remains unstable and the patient complains of it giving way. Complex multiple ligament injuries are usually treated by combined surgical repair and reconstruction, but there is often persistent instability when knee movements are regained.

The treatment of chronic ligamentous instability of the knee has become a specialized field involving accurate diagnosis and multiple reconstructive procedures. The majority of surgeons in the UK use autograft (graft from the patient) for simple cruciate surgery, the two most commonly used sources being the hamstring tendons and the patella ligament. For more complex procedures with multiple ligaments injured, the surgeon will often use allograft (donor tissue) to save time and morbidity associated with taking grafts. Anchoring the graft to bone sufficiently to allow early stressing presents some problems, but the long-term aim is for the graft to be re-vascularized and, in effect, to form a new ligament. In order to do this, some controlled longitudinal stress appears to be important. The repair can be carried out arthroscopically, which makes early mobilization much easier.

Fractures of the patella

These common fractures are of two types.

Comminuted fracture

This type of fracture is caused by a direct blow, often against the dashboard of a car. There is likely to be damage to the underlying femoral condyles (Fig. 22.2).

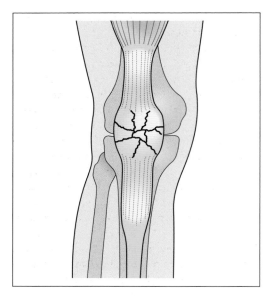

Figure 22.2 Comminuted stellate fracture of the patella.

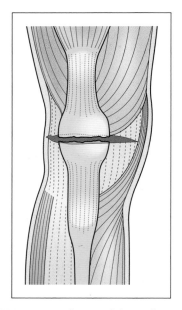

Figure 22.3 Transverse fracture of the patella.

Treatment

Surgery is advised to reduce and fix the fracture. This can be very difficult, but excising the patella should be avoided if possible. Rehabilitation depends partly on how stable the fracture is after fixation. Early movement is the gold standard and physiotherapy is needed to mobilize the knee and regain quadriceps power.

Avulsion or transverse fracture

This is caused by violent contraction of the quadriceps against resistance. The patella is frequently torn in two horizontally, and the split extends laterally into the quadriceps expansion (Fig. 22.3).

Treatment

Open reduction is carried out and the position held with a figure-of-eight wire. Early mobilization is possible after stable fixation to avoid stiffness and muscle atrophy.

A late complication following any patellar fracture may be osteoarthritis of the patellofemoral compartment.

Rupture of the quadriceps tendon

The same mechanism which causes a transverse fracture of the patella may also result in a transverse rupture of the quadriceps tendon just above the patella. These injuries tend to occur in middle age and are often overlooked by inexperienced casualty doctors. The patient is unable to straight-leg raise and there is a palpable gap in the tendon. If there is any doubt an ultrasound scan can confirm the diagnosis.

Treatment

Surgical repair is advised, followed by a period of immobilization and rehabilitation with physiotherapy.

Rupture of patella ligament

This injury differs from a quadriceps rupture in that it tends to occur in younger, more athletic individuals who may have a history of patella tendinosis. Usually clinically obvious, an X-ray will show a high patella. The patient is unable to straight-leg raise and tenderness is present below the patella.

Treatment

Surgical repair is necessary and if a circlage wire is also used, early mobilization is possible.

Fractures of the tibia and fibula

Fractures of the upper tibia

Fractures of the intercondylar region are avulsion injuries and have been mentioned in connection with the anterior cruciate ligament. Fractures of the tibial plateau are usually caused by a forcible valgus or varus strain, e.g. by being struck by a car bumper (Fig. 22.4). The knee fills with blood and may feel unstable on lateral and medial stressing. These injuries most commonly affect the lateral tibial plateau but can be medial or both. Fractures of both medial and lateral sides of the plateau are high-energy injuries and are very difficult to treat, requiring specialist input.

Simple stable fractures can be treated conservatively in a brace to encourage movement.

Displaced fractures, where there is significant disruption of the joint surface, are better treated by open elevation of the joint surface with a bone graft to fill the underlying defect. Plates and screws hold the fracture whilst it heals. In some cases the procedure can be carried out arthroscopically. Mobilization should be encouraged as early as possible to avoid stiffness, and a cast-brace is useful to provide protection when the patient leaves hospital. Very severe fractures on both sides of the knee can be treated with circular frames (external fixator) or with newer designs of 'locking' plates. Care must be taken and surgery planned to avoid infection. A late complication is osteoarthritis.

Fractures of the tibial shaft and fibula

These are extremely common injuries in all age groups and are frequently open, sometimes with a very extensive and contaminated wound. They often follow road traffic and sporting accidents. Diagnosis is usually obvious. The X-ray gives some indication of the mechanism of injury and of the likely stability of the fracture after reduction. Oblique and spiral fractures of the tibia are usually unstable after reduction. If the fibula is not fractured, closed reduction of the fracture of the tibia may be difficult and if in these circumstances conservative treatment is adopted, there is always a tendency for the tibial fracture to displace into a varus position. Internal fixation may be preferred.

Treatment

Wound management is all-important in securing early union of open fractures. The wound is treated with aggressive early debridement and closed as quickly as possible, though rarely immediately. Grossly contaminated wounds are usually best left open after removal of all necrotic and foreign material. Plastic surgical techniques, using rotated or free full-thickness grafts with vascular anastomosis, often incorporating muscle, have become important in achieving early soft-tissue healing (see Chapter 2, p. 13).

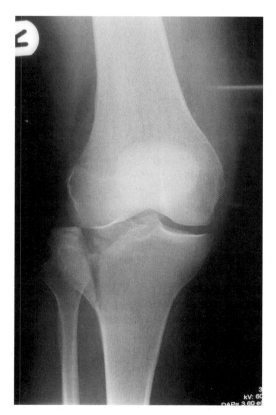

Figure 22.4 Fracture of the tibial plateau.

Transverse tibial shaft fractures are reasonably stable when reduced, with little tendency to shorten. They can usually be held in a well-fitting full leg plaster-cast with the knee flexed to 20–30 degrees to prevent rotation at the fracture site. If the tibial fracture is spiral or comminuted, some means must be found to prevent shortening. A full leg plaster-cast alone is rarely sufficient. There are many possibilities and the choice will often depend on available resources and facilities.

1 Internal fixation has become the most popular choice for most unstable tibial fractures, its proponents claiming earlier mobilization, more certain union and better alignment. Plating, usually with a compression plate, has been widely used, but has now largely given way to intramedullary nailing, particularly with a locked nail (Fig. 22.5). The complication rate, however, can be high with any form of internal fixation and infection is a constant risk, particularly if the fracture is open. Considerable expertise is needed to obtain consistently good results from internal fixation and if this is lacking or theatre facilities are poor, conservative management is often the safer option.

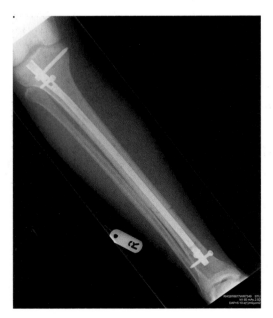

Figure 22.5 Locked nail for tibial fracture.

2 Internal fixation carries particular risks if the fracture is associated with an extensive or badly contaminated wound. In these circumstances, **external frame fixation**, with pins placed above and below the fracture (see Fig. 5.14), gives good fixation and allows access to the wound for dressing, grafting, etc. This type of fracture is often slow to unite and union may be further inhibited by rigid fixation. Frames which allow controlled mobility of the fracture in the early stages may prove better in this respect.

3 Conservative treatment usually relies on plaster-cast fixation.

4 A close-fitting cast-brace which allows knee movement (Sarmiento) can give good results, but needs considerable expertise. Weight-bearing is permitted after 3 weeks.

Length of treatment

The time it takes for a tibial shaft fracture to heal depends on a number of factors. High-energy, open fractures or those complicated by compartment syndrome take longer to heal. Patients who smoke and older patients may also progress to union more slowly. Opinions vary as to when weight-bearing should be started. Most conservatively treated tibial fractures require at least 3 months' immobilization and may take 5 or more months to unite. If the fracture is stable, particularly after intramedullary nailing or circular frame fixation, weight-bearing can be started almost immediately. In other cases it is usually delayed for at least 6 weeks.

Isolated fractures of the fibular shaft

These are of little significance, and can be treated with a supportive dressing or plaster-cast until painless.

Complications of lower limb fractures

1 Non-union of tibial fractures is common, especially when complicated by infection.
2 Some degree of ischaemia of the deep muscles of the calf (compartment syndrome) is common and may result in the patient developing flexion contractures of the toes.

3 Stiffness of knee, ankle and foot may delay full rehabilitation.

Meniscal injuries

Meniscus lesions

The menisci are the fibro-cartilaginous 'shock absorbers' of the knee, attached firmly at either end to the tibial eminence (Fig. 22.6). They have a loose attachment to the capsule around their peripheries where vessels enter the meniscus. Tears through this area have the potential for healing.

The medial meniscus is more circular and the lateral C-shaped. As the lateral meniscus is mobile it can move away from potential injury. The medial meniscus is more fixed and twice as likely to be torn.

Discoid meniscus

In early embryonic life, both menisci form a complete septum between the tibia and femur. They normally develop a central opening well before birth. Rarely, one of them remains as a complete disc. This normally affects the lateral meniscus. It is often discovered during childhood or early adult life because of its tendency to 'clunk' loudly as the joint moves. It is more liable to tear than the normal meniscus and the tear may be the cause of symptoms. The condition is frequently asymptomatic and never discovered, but if it causes trouble the meniscus may be excised.

Tears of the menisci

These are some of the commonest knee injuries. It is likely that many menisci which tear are degenerate, particularly in older patients.

Typical features

The patient, normally a young male, twists the knee whilst it is flexed and the weight is on that leg. He/she feels something tear and experiences pain on the side of the knee where the meniscus is torn. The knee may lock, i.e. extension may be impossible. Occasionally, the knee may be manipulated causing it to 'unlock' suddenly. The footballer is usually not able to carry on playing. The knee swells, usually over the next 6–12 hours. Occasionally, swelling occurs within 15–30 minutes. This is due to a haemarthrosis and may mean a cruciate or synovial tear, either of which may be associated with a meniscus tear.

The typical course is then for the swelling and pain to subside over the next few days and for the knee gradually to regain full extension.

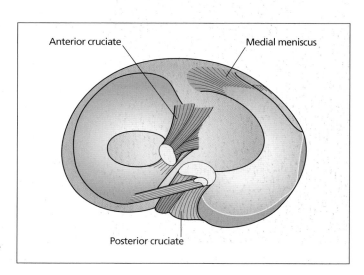

Figure 22.6 The menisci and cruciate ligaments at the knee.

Occasionally, the joint remains locked and the swelling and pain persist. After 12–14 days the knee may appear to be back to normal. Symptoms may then recur if the knee is provoked, e.g. by football or a twisting strain at work. It may then lock intermittently, 'give way' due to reflex quadriceps inhibition, and cause episodes of pain and swelling. The pain may move from its original site, causing diagnostic difficulties. The anterior cruciate and medial ligaments are frequently damaged together with the medial meniscus, causing instability of the joint.

The clinical picture is frequently much less classical than that described above, and a tear may occur with minimal violence, particularly in individuals who spend much time crouching. In these cases it is often the persistence of symptoms which leads to the diagnosis.

Signs

At the time of the original injury there may be swelling, tenderness over the meniscus, muscle spasm and perhaps loss of full extension. In the chronic state, the only signs may be wasting of the quadriceps, perhaps a moderate effusion and usually tenderness over the appropriate joint line. The patient rarely tolerates a locked knee for long.

Pathology (Fig. 22.7)

1 The commonest tear runs longitudinally along the cartilage, separating a central 'bucket-handle' fragment from a lateral fragment, which is still attached peripherally. This bucket-handle varies in thickness and may represent the whole width of the meniscus, when it is called a peripheral detachment.

2 The peripheral detachment may only affect the anterior or posterior horns.

3 Also common is a horizontal cleavage tear, which may produce a flap which catches between the condyles ('parrot beak' tear).

Diagnosis

If an accurate clinical diagnosis of a meniscus tear is to be made, the patient should either have a classical history or classical physical signs or preferably both. Many patients are atypical and can present difficult diagnostic problems. The commonest conditions to be confused with a meniscus tear are ligamentous strains, osteochondritis dissecans, osteoarthritis and acute synovitis. Even at arthroscopy, some patients with a good history and physical signs are found to have no obvious pathology.

Investigations

An ordinary X-ray is only of value in confirming or excluding other conditions. MRI scanning is the investigation of choice if there is doubt about the diagnosis.

Arthroscopy is a well-established technique. It gives an excellent view of most of the structures in the joint, including the posterior half of the menisci, which are not visible through an anterior surgical incision (Fig. 22.8).

Meniscectomy

Arthroscopic surgery is now so well-established that almost all meniscus surgery is carried out

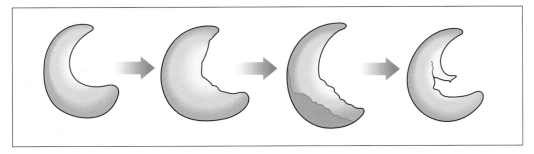

Figure 22.7 Pathology of tears of the meniscus.

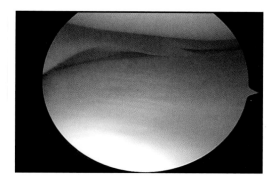

Figure 22.8 Arthroscopic view of a torn meniscus.

arthroscopically. Special instruments have been devised to carry out the operative manoeuvres through small puncture wounds and under direct arthroscopic vision. The joint is not opened and recovery from the surgery can be much more rapid than with conventional open techniques. There is evidence that osteoarthritis may follow excision of a normal meniscus, and it certainly follows a proportion of meniscectomies for a torn meniscus. Current opinion favours trying to preserve as much of the meniscus as possible by trimming away damaged fragments and, wherever possible, repairing longitudinal peripheral tears.

Cyst of the menisci

A cyst usually arises from the lateral meniscus and enlarges under the capsule, forming a swelling which is tense in certain positions of flexion. It is accurately located over the meniscus and does not usually reach a large size. It may give rise to pain from tension, and the meniscus, which is usually degenerate and filled with a honeycomb of cysts, is liable to tear, producing acute or chronic symptoms. Removal of the torn meniscus is more likely to produce a lasting cure than simple removal of the cyst.

Inflammatory conditions (see Chapter 10)

Rheumatoid arthritis usually affects the knee, causing pain, stiffness, synovial thickening and effusion. Joint destruction can be very severe and

may lead to secondary osteoarthritis, treated frequently by TKR. The usual medical and supportive treatment regimes often control the disease in the knee. Every attempt should be made to retain movements. If instability becomes a problem, a removable splint may be helpful in maintaining the patient's mobility.

Ankylosing spondylitis

This may cause a similar arthritis to that in rheumatoid arthritis.

Gout

This commonly affects the knee, usually on one side only. Severe pain and effusion occur in attacks and are usually controlled by rest and drug therapy.

Degenerative conditions (see Chapter 11)

Popliteal cysts

These are common at all ages and usually present as painless swellings in the popliteal fossa, often fluctuating in size. They may arise from one of the anatomical bursae. They tend to be placed medially and rarely reach a large size. They need only be excised if they are giving rise to symptoms. Larger and more diffuse cysts are often associated with pathology in the knee joint, particularly rheumatoid and, less commonly, osteoarthritis. These invariably have a direct connection with the back of the joint through a small defect in the capsule. The rheumatoid cysts are particularly liable to extend and may infiltrate the calf muscles. They are often known as 'Baker's cysts'.

Treatment

The cyst itself is usually of less consequence than the associated arthritis. If a synovectomy is to be carried out this will often cause the cyst to disappear. Extensive cysts may cause pain and interfere with function and may need to be dissected out, but this can be a difficult procedure. The differential diagnosis of popliteal aneurysm should always be considered.

Osteoarthritis

The knee is one of the commonest joints to be affected by osteoarthritis. It is common in patients with lower limb deformity. In a valgus knee (knock knee), more weight is carried through the lateral compartment and the patellofemoral joint (Fig. 22.9). With a varus knee (bow leg), the weight is greatest through the medial compartment.

Other predisposing conditions are fractures, infective conditions, meniscus and ligamentous injuries, osteochondritis dissecans and rheumatoid arthritis.

Pathology

The knee shows the typical pathological features of extensive wearing away of joint cartilage, with fraying of the menisci, marginal osteophytes and some synovial thickening, but little inflammatory reaction. X-rays show the typical features of loss of joint space, cyst, sclerosis and osteophytes (Fig. 22.10).

Treatment

Many patients can be managed adequately by conservative methods, e.g. by losing weight, using a stick, modifying their work, taking analgesics and non-steroidal anti-inflammatory agents as necessary, with physiotherapy in the form of heat and exercises in an attempt to maintain range and quadriceps power.

Surgery

A large number of patients still have symptoms severe enough to warrant surgery. The possibilities are:

1 Arthroscopic lavage/debridement. This is controversial and is probably no better than conservative treatment in severe arthritis. It may have a limited role in mild osteoarthritis.

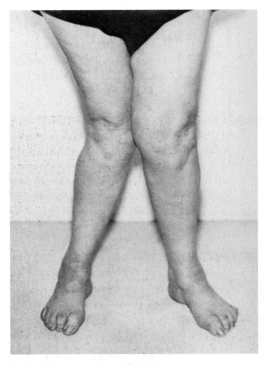

Figure 22.9 Valgus deformity of the knee leading to osteoarthritis.

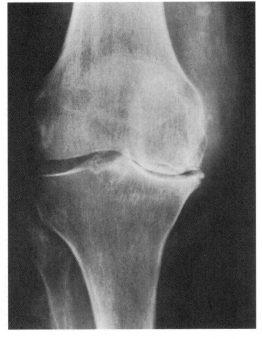

Figure 22.10 X-ray appearance of osteoarthritis of the knee.

2 Arthrodesis. This is used very rarely now as joint replacement has taken its place. It is occasionally used for failed knee replacements. It gives good pain relief but patients do not like having a stiff knee as this makes sitting awkward.

3 Osteotomy. This still has a role in younger patients, particularly heavy manual workers. The aim is to correct the abnormal alignment to allow the normal side of the knee to take more load.

4 Arthroplasty. Knee replacement is by far the most common operation for knee osteoarthritis. The replacement can be either of the whole joint—total knee replacement (TKR) or part of it—uni-compartmental knee replacement (UKR). Only some knees are suitable for UKR. Total replacement is often the procedure of choice and many different types are available mostly giving good results for at least 10 years.

Present techniques concentrate on two basic designs:

• Unconstrained type which is essentially a lining for the condyles and relies on the joint's own ligaments for stability.

• Partly constrained type, which has some inherent stability, usually dependent on the shape of the articular surfaces (Fig. 22.11).

Infections (see Chapter 13)

Acute infections

The upper end of the tibia and the lower end of the femur are the commonest sites for acute osteomyelitis in children (see Chapter 13, p. 102). Spread of infection to the joint is uncommon.

Acute suppurative arthritis is usually seen either in neonates or in adults suffering from rheumatoid arthritis and on steroid therapy. In this latter circumstance the inflammatory response may be considerably masked by the steroids.

Acute arthritis of the knee in a young adult may be due to gonorrhoeal infection.

Treatment of all infective conditions around the knee is aided by immobilization of the joint.

Chronic infections

Tuberculosis of the knee is rare in Europe, but still common in under-developed areas. It is characterized by chronic pain and swelling, usually with severe muscle wasting. The condition is usually recognized and treatment instituted before serious destruction occurs, and with modern antibiotic therapy a useful joint may be preserved.

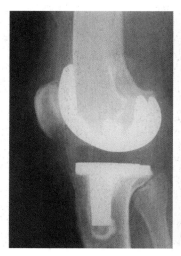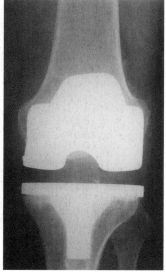

Figure 22.11 Knee prosthesis *in situ*.

Neoplastic conditions (see Chapter 12)

Metastatic neoplasms are common in both the tibia and femur and may result in pain in the knee.

Primary neoplasms of bone are very rare but should always be in the back of the physician's mind. Certain features (red flags) alert the clinician, such as atypical pain, night pain, no history of injury, and mass or swelling in a young patient. The upper end of the tibia and fibula and lower end of the femur are the commonest sites for several tumours, notably osteosarcoma and osteoclastoma. They usually present as a painful swelling and may cause a sympathetic effusion in the joint.

Metabolic diseases of the knee (see Chapter 14)

Few metabolic diseases cause specific problems at the knee. Genu valgum or genu varum may occur as a result of rickets or renal rickets. Scurvy may result in subperiosteal haematoma in the tibia. Paget's disease typically causes thickening and bowing of the tibia, often with pseudofractures. Pathological fractures are common in the tibia and osteoarthritis may occur in the knee joint affected by Paget's disease.

Loose bodies

These tend to cause symptoms by becoming trapped between the joint surfaces. Locking or giving way is usual and the body may be palpable. Loose bodies containing articular cartilage may gradually increase in size.

The knee is the commonest joint to develop loose bodies. These may result from:
1 Osteochondritis dissecans
2 Osteochondral fractures
3 Detached osteophytes, usually in osteoarthritis
4 Soft-tissue fragments, e.g. from a damaged meniscus
5 Synovial chondromatosis is a rare condition where the whole synovium may be studded with cartilaginous nodules. One or more may break free into the joint.

Treatment

A loose body which is causing symptoms should usually be removed using the arthroscope or, if necessary, by open operation.

Chapter 23

The foot and ankle

Patients with foot and ankle problems make up a considerable proportion of those attending primary care and hospitals. Problems usually are related to pain, deformity or loss of function, or most often a combination of all three.

Functional anatomy

Knowledge of the anatomy of the foot and ankle is key to understanding the disorders which present. The ankle joint is more complex than a simple hinge. Most of the body weight is transmitted from the tibia through the talus. The fibula also plays a part in weight-bearing through its articulation with the talus. The tibia and fibula are held firmly together by strong ligaments at the knee and at the ankle (Fig. 23.1).

On the medial side of the ankle, the deltoid ligament is a broad structure running from the tip of the medial malleolus distally to the talus, navicular and calcaneus in a fan shape.

On the lateral side, the lateral ligament complex consists of three bands, the anterior talofibular ligament (ATFL), the calcaneofibular ligament (CFL) and the posterior talofibular ligament (PTFL). Sprains of the ankle usually affect the ATFL, but a

more severe injury may involve all three, rendering the ankle unstable (Fig. 23.2).

The subtalar joint lies between the talus and the calcaneum and provides for inversion and eversion of the heel. The talonavicular and calcaneocuboid joints (together known as Chopart's joint) also act with the subtalar joint to allow pronation and supination movements of the foot.

The plantar calcaneonavicular ligament, also known as the 'spring' ligament, suspends the head of the talus and together with the long plantar ligament and the plantar aponeurosis contribute to maintaining the medial longitudinal arch of the foot.

The hindfoot and midfoot joints are coupled in a complex manner such that the lower the medial longitudinal arch (flat foot or pes planus deformity), the more the forefoot tends to be abducted. An abnormally high arch is called pes cavus and is often associated with an adducted forefoot. During normal standing and walking, pressure is taken on the heel, the lateral foot and the heads of all the metatarsals (look at your wet foot print on a dry floor to see this).

The intercuneiform and the tarsometatarsal joints each allow a little gliding movement and are important to the overall flexibility of the foot and its ability to accommodate to uneven terrain.

Considering the foot more distally, the first metatarsophalangeal joint (MTPJ) has two small,

Lecture Notes: Orthopaedics and Fractures, 4e.
By T Duckworth and CM Blundell. Published 2010 by Blackwell Publishing.

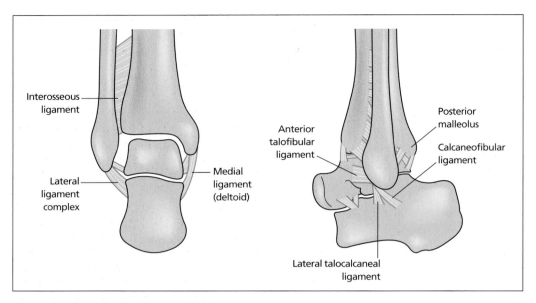

Figure 23.1 Ligaments supporting the ankle.

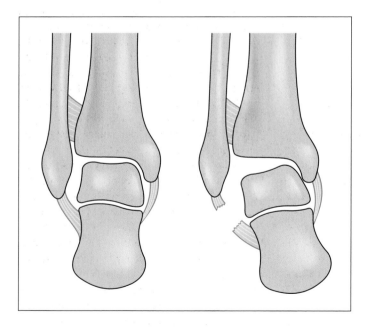

Figure 23.2 Lateral ligament rupture renders the ankle unstable.

but important bones (sesamoids) which lie within the flexor hallucis brevis tendon beneath the head of the first metatarsal. These take much of the body weight, 70% of which is taken by the big toe with each foot step. The first MTPJ is a frequent source of pain and deformity. Dorsiflexion of the MTPJs is important in the 'push-off' movement of normal walking.

Box 23.1 Summary of foot and ankle examination.

Look	Deformity
	Gait
	Wasting
	Swelling
Feel	Tenderness
	Temperature
Movements	Isolate each joint 'system in turn
Neurology	Especially sensory, but also motor
Circulation	DP, PT and capillary refill

Examination (see also Box 23.1)

1 Look:

Gait. Normal gait is made up of a stance phase (the foot on the floor) and a swing phase (the foot off the floor). Gait assessment is complex and it takes a well trained eye to unravel an abnormal gait into its constituent parts, let alone make a diagnosis! Some simple abnormalities of gait are:

- A painful or *antalgic gait* is characterized by putting the foot down as lightly and for as little time as possible (a short stance phase) and is the commonest reason for a 'limp'
- A stiff or painful ankle results in external rotation of the affected limb when walking
- Paralysis of dorsiflexion (a foot drop) results in a characteristic high stepping gait to get the foot clear during the swing phase.

Deformity. Each section of the foot should be considered independently when assessing deformities and movement. The patient should be assessed initially whilst standing.

- *The hindfoot in its relationship to the tibia:*
  1 When looked at from behind with the patient weight-bearing, the heel may be in line with the tibia or may be inclined inwards—*varus*, or outwards—*valgus*. Normal alignment is around 5 degrees of valgus
  2 When looked at from the side, the long axis of the calcaneum normally inclines upwards and forwards (Fig. 23.3). If this line is inclined more downwards than normal, the position is called *equinus*, and if more upwards than normal *calcaneus*.

- *The forefoot in its relationship to the hindfoot:*
  1 Normally aligned
  2 Dorsiflexed or plantarflexed
  3 Adducted or abducted or
  4 Rotated (supinated or pronated).
- *The toes in their relationship to the metatarsals and in the joints within the toes.*

Wasting. The muscles of the calf and anterior compartment may show wasting in foot and ankle disease. Wasting of the peroneal muscles on the lateral side of the leg occurs in several neurological conditions.

Swelling. Swelling of the ankle and foot is often due to oedema which 'pits' on pressure. This may be due to generalized disease or to a local condition. Discrete swellings should be described in the usual way and their relationship to weight-bearing and pressure from the shoe noted. On the sole of the foot, thickened skin (callosities) should be noted and its relationship to the metatarsal heads recorded.

Remember to always inspect the sole of the foot as well as between the toes. Ulcers and swellings can be surprisingly easily overlooked otherwise.

2 Feel. The main bony landmarks should be palpated. Tenderness and temperature should be accurately assessed. The foot and toes are frequently cold in neurological and circulatory conditions. Increased temperature occurs in inflammatory conditions, such as infections, gout and rheumatoid arthritis. Assessment of pulses and sensation are often included at this stage.

3 Movements. Ankle movements are tested by flexing the whole foot in the ankle mortice with the subtalar joint held in neutral. Fifty degrees of plantarflexion and 20–30 degrees of dorsiflexion are normal. There is normally no varus or valgus movement at the ankle joint, but varus may occur if the lateral ligaments are disrupted.

Subtalar movements are tested by holding the heel and gliding it from side to side on the talus. Inversion and eversion are complex coupled movements involving the subtalar and Chopart's joints together.

Mid-tarsal movements are tested by grasping the heel firmly to hold it still and rotating the midfoot around the hindfoot. Movements are usually

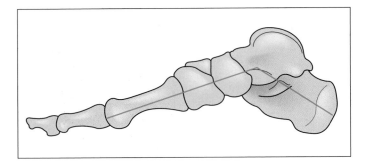

Figure 23.3 Position of the normal calcaneum.

restricted to a few degrees of rotation, which is partly mid-tarsal and partly intertarsal.

The metatarsals can be moved slightly on the tarsus at the Lisfranc's joint.

Toe movements are tested individually at each joint.

Many of these movements may be painful, so care must be taken and the patient's face must be observed for signs of discomfort during the examination.

4 Neurology. A careful neurological assessment is always necessary because of the close relationship between foot pathology and many systemic conditions, such as diabetes, which is the commonest cause of a sensory neuropathy. Many congenital deformities have a neurological aetiology.

5 Circulation. Assessment of the circulation is vital both for diagnosis and to guide treatment. The dorsalis pedis (DP) and posterior tibial (PT) pulses should be recorded, as should capillary refill time. A sore on the tip of the toe or incipient gangrene is a frequent sign of peripheral vascular disease.

Congenital conditions

Congenital conditions affecting the foot and ankle are dealt with in Chapter 8.

Developmental conditions

Flat foot

Most cases of flat foot (pes planus) in children are physiological. More severe pes planus is usually associated with paralytic conditions, such as cere-

bral palsy in children. In teenagers and young adults, congenital abnormalities of the hindfoot, particularly congenital partial fusions between the hindfoot bones (tarsal coalitions), present quite late.

Pes cavus

In the normal foot, the long axis of the calcaneum runs upwards and forwards (Fig. 23.3). The longitudinal arch may be abnormally high irrespective of the attitude of the heel, though most often the heel is in varus (cavovarus foot). Severe degrees of pes cavus are usually associated with clawing of the toes (Fig. 23.4) and are often secondary to a neurological condition (such as spina bifida or polio), with weakness of the interossei. The effects on the foot are similar to interosseus weakness in the hands.

In some of these conditions there may be sensory loss and this, coupled with the deformity, may result in pressure ulcers developing under the metatarsal heads or on the outer border of the foot.

Severe clawing of the toes not infrequently results in dislocation of the MTPJs.

Treatment of claw toes

If the deformity can be passively corrected (flexible), then transplanting the long flexor tendon around the side of the toe into the extensor tendon may correct the position (Girdlestone). If the deformity is fixed, then the proximal interphalangeal joint usually is fused and the extensor tendon divided. The dislocated MTPJ may require shortening of the metatarsal (Weil osteotomy) or partial

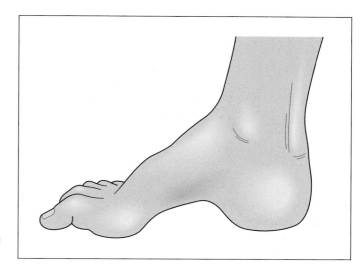

Figure 23.4 Pes cavus and clawing of the toes.

excision of the proximal phalanx (Stainsby procedure) to produce adequate correction.

The pes cavus may require a combination of soft-tissue and bony surgery to correct the deformity and rebalance the foot.

Hallux valgus

This is a condition in which the first metatarsal deviates medially to a variable degree (metatarsus primus varus) and the great toe deviates laterally and may be rotated into pronation. This results in a medial prominence (a bunion) at the first MTPJ.

It is often associated with elevation of the first metatarsal, causing a loss of the transverse arch and subsequent overload of the lateral metatarsals (so-called transfer metatarsalgia). The big toe may cross over or under the second toe (Fig. 23.5). Hammer toe deformity, especially of the second toe, is commonly associated with this condition.

Clinical features

The condition is much more common in women. The aetiology is unknown. There is no definite evidence that it is caused by unsuitable footwear, but the pain is exacerbated by badly fitting shoes. It may start in late childhood or early adult life, and

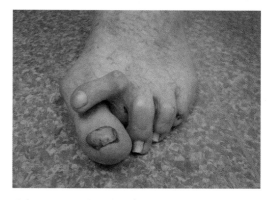

Figure 23.5 Hallux vagus showing crossing over of the second toe.

usually progresses. The first MTPJ usually remains mobile, but due to the deformity, the great toe ceases to take load effectively during walking.

The prominent medial exostosis, which is usually present, aches and sometimes an adventitious bursa may form under the skin overlying the prominent metatarsal head. This may become acutely inflamed and painful.

Treatment

Many patients are asymptomatic but may need to select their shoes carefully. Metatarsalgia may be helped by wearing a metatarsal support which fits in the shoe and supports the metatarsal necks on a cushion, relieving pressure on the heads.

Surgery may be necessary in some patients. Many procedures are available. A few of the more common are listed below.

1 Metatarsal osteotomy. There have been many first metatarsal osteotomies described. An osteotomy which is widely used currently is the Scarf osteotomy. This is a Z-shaped osteotomy which allows correction of the metatarsal deformity in three planes (Fig. 23.6). It is stable and can be tailored to suit the individual deformity, hence its popularity. Scarf osteotomy is often combined with a corrective procedure to the proximal phalanx (Akin osteotomy). This retains joint movement and restores function to the first ray.

2 Arthrodesis (fusion) of the metatarsophalangeal joint. If in addition to the deformity there is established osteoarthritis of the first MTPJ, the fusion will result in correction of the deformity and resolution of pain. Providing the fusion is carried out in the correct position it gives good long-term function, but in women it may restrict the height of heel which can be worn on the shoe.

The great toe still takes part in weight-bearing after a metatarsophalangeal fusion.

Traumatic conditions

The ankle is a stable joint, with congruent bony surfaces and strong ligamentous support.

Ligament injuries

These are the commonest ankle injuries by far. The anterior talofibular ligament (ATFL) is usually sprained or the ligament may be ruptured by 'going over' on the outside of the foot, i.e. an inversion stress often accompanied by a twisting component. More severe sprains involve other lateral ligaments or rarely the deltoid ligament on the medial side.

Clinical features

The ankle is swollen and painful with restriction of movements and tenderness localized over the lateral ligament. When an attempt is made to invert the foot, there is pain and muscle spasm in the peronei. Differentiation from a fracture of the lateral malleolus is difficult and X-rays may be needed, guided by the Ottowa ankle rules which have a

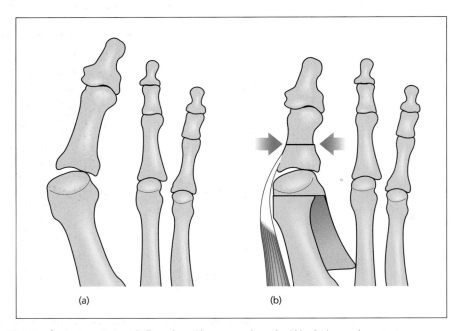

(a)   (b)

Figure 23.6 Scarf osteotomy to treat hallux valgus. Blue arrows show the Akin closing wedge osteotomy.

sensitivity for ankle fracture of almost 100%. The Ottawa ankle rules have been developed specifically for determining which ankle injuries require X-ray. They relate to sites of pain at the fifth metatarsal base and navicular and an inability to weight-bear.

Treatment

1 A simple sprain can be protected by strapping or, if the ankle is very swollen, by a below-knee walking cast for 2–3 weeks.

2 If the signs are severe, and particularly if the ankle is swollen on both sides, complete rupture should be suspected and treated accordingly. MRI scanning may confirm this, though its reliability has been questioned. It may, however, show an occult fracture or an injury to the tibiofibular syndesmosis. A complete rupture may be treated conservatively, as there is no good evidence to confirm that operative treatment is superior. A weight-bearing below-knee cast may be used for 6 weeks. Alternatively, early mobilization may be allowed, provided the ligament is protected by a suitable brace. An inadequately treated rupture may result in persistent instability, with the joint tending to give way during normal use.

3 Long-term instability, with opening of the joint on stressing, may require surgical reconstruction of the lateral ligament either by direct repair (so called 'anatomic repair') or using the peroneus brevis tendon (a 'non-anatomic repair').

4 Medial ligament sprains are uncommon but should be taken seriously as a complete rupture carries a poor prognosis without operative repair.

Fractures and dislocations of the ankle

Classification

Many fractures of the ankle are associated with subluxation or dislocation of the joint surfaces. The variety of such injuries is wide and many classifications have been attempted. Most of these are based on speculation as to the precise mechanism by which the injury has been caused, and none can be regarded as entirely satisfactory in covering all the possibilities. Those commonly used are a simple description of which malleoli have been fractured, the Weber classification and the Lauge–Hansen classification.

Simple description

The subject can be simplified by understanding that the joint can be injured on one side only (single malleolus; Fig. 23.7) or on both sides

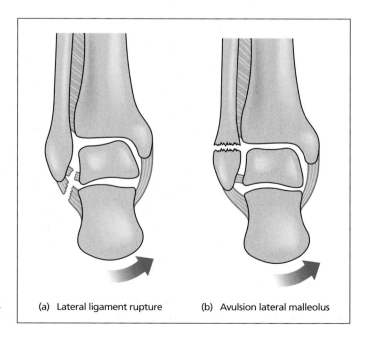

Figure 23.7 Uni-malleolar injuries, sustained by adduction.

(a) Lateral ligament rupture   (b) Avulsion lateral malleolus

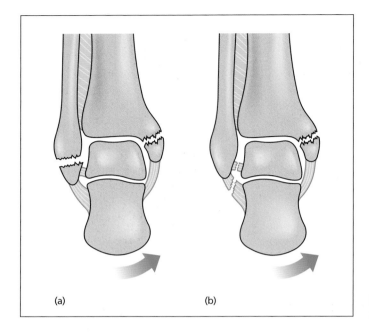

(a)   (b)

Figure 23.8 Bi-malleolar injuries, sustained by adduction.

(bi-malleolar fracture; Fig. 23.8). In rotational injuries, one or both sides may be injured, as well as the posterior lip of the lower end of the tibia, which is fractured by the talus as it rotates out of the ankle (Fig. 23.9c). This structure is often called the posterior malleolus and may prove to be key in treating these injuries operatively.

The degree of instability depends on how much of the ankle complex is damaged. A minimally displaced single malleolar fracture may be managed in a cast or brace (usually the lateral malleolus). If there has been a shift of the talus in the ankle joint, then this must be reduced with a manipulation or with surgery. A bi-malleolar fracture is often associated with shift of the talus and is best managed with open reduction and internal fixation (ORIF) in order to restore the articular anatomy and provide stability. Tri-malleolar fractures should be operatively managed. Table 23.1 is to be used as a guide only.

Weber classification
It has been convincingly demonstrated that when a patient 'goes over' forcibly with his/her full weight on the ankle, the violent inversion of the foot is converted by the oblique direction of the subtalar joint into a force causing the talus to rotate outwards in the ankle mortice ('torque convertor' mechanism). It is the talus attempting to rotate externally within the fixed ankle mortice which causes this type of fracture. A rotational force appears to cause various types of injury with combinations of fractures and ligament damage. An important structure in maintaining ankle stability is the strong interosseous ligament between the lower ends of the tibia and fibula; the distal tibio-fibular syndesmosis. Fractures can be subdivided into those where this ligament is intact (syndesmosis intact) and those in which it is completely ruptured (a distasis of the syndesmosis).

This is the basis of the Weber classification of ankle injuries, which is simple and helps to guide management and is thus widely used (Fig. 23.10). Unfortunately it only formally takes account of the lateral malleolus fracture, although injury medially, either to the deltoid ligament or malleolus, can be inferred. A summary is given in Table 23.2.

Lauge–Hansen classification
This system is more complex but, because of its completeness, is a frequently-used classification (it was devised in 1950). It uses two terms—the first

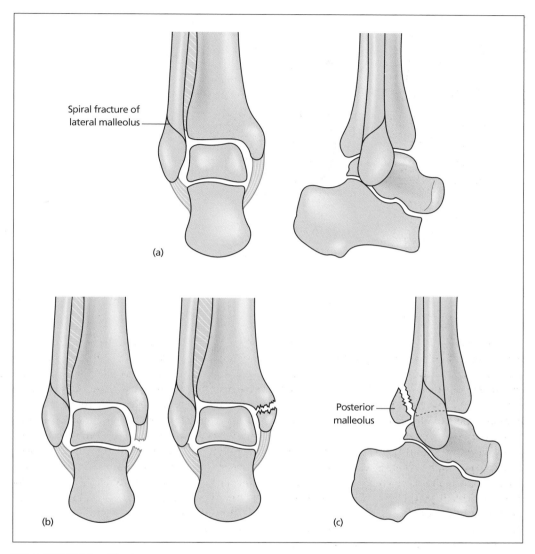

Figure 23.9 Rotational fractures.

describes the position of the foot at the time of the injury and the second the motion of the talus relative to the tibia.

1 Supination—adduction
2 Supination—external rotation
3 Pronation—abduction
4 Pronation—eversion
5 Pronation—dorsiflexion.

This description is used because most ankle injuries are caused by the weight of the falling person applying a force to the ankle with the foot in a fixed position. The classification proposes that the mechanism of injury can be deduced from the X-ray appearances and that reduction involves applying the reverse movement.

It should be emphasized that this classification is based on the static X-ray appearances. There is considerable inter-observer error in classifying the injuries and there is much to be said for simply analysing each fracture in terms of the degree and

Table 23.1 Simple guide to ankle fracture management.

Description	Displacement of talus	Treatment
Single malleolus	No	Cast or brace 6 weeks
	Yes	Reduce non-operatively or open reduction and internal fixation (ORIF)
Bi-malleolar	Likely	ORIF
Tri-malleolar	Likely	ORIF

direction of instability. The details of the Lauge–Hansen classification are beyond the scope of this book.

Treatment

The evidence suggests that anatomical reduction of the fractures, with accurate location of the talus within the ankle mortice, gives the best results and that the technique of maintaining reduction is less important. In practice, internal fixation is often the easiest way of maintaining the position, but it is by no means always necessary.

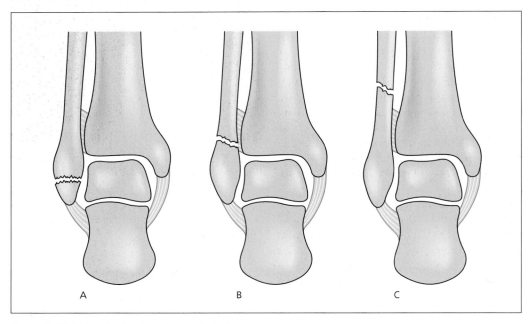

Figure 23.10 Weber classification of uni-malleolar fractures.

Table 23.2 Lateral malleolus fractures.

Weber classification	Level of fracture	Displacement	Management
A	Below syndesmosis	None usually	Bandage or cast weight-bearing
B	At syndesmosis	If none, usually medial side uninjured If displaced, often medial side is injured	Cast weight-bearing Open reduction and internal fixation of fracture
C	Above syndesmosis	Suggests medial injury also	Reduce syndesmosis injury

A special note must be made for ankle fractures in patients with diabetes. In diabetics bones heal more slowly and patients often have a degree of peripheral sensory neuropathy. These fractures *must* be immobilized for twice the normal period used for non-diabetics as these patients are prone to delayed union and skin breakdown. Charcot arthropathy must always been borne in mind.

1 Uni-malleolar. These have some intrinsic stability and can usually be controlled with a bandage or light-weight malleolar splint. Sometimes a plaster-cast is needed, particularly if the pain is too great in a compression bandage. Six weeks' weight-bearing immobilization is usually sufficient.

2 Bi-malleolar injuries. These are unstable in several planes. They can sometimes be adequately held in a plaster-cast, particularly if the medial malleolus is partly intact. In most cases, internal fixation will be needed and usually a contoured plate and screws are used. Higher fibular fractures (Weber C injuries, see Table 23.2) can be fixed in the same way, with good control of ankle stability. The deltoid ligament need not be repaired, but a medial fragment (unless tiny), is best re-attached with a pair of parallel screws or a tension-band wire.

If the interosseous ligament is ruptured, then this must be addressed by stabilizing this joint with a horizontal screw (a diastasis screw) orientated in the inter-malleolar plane. If such a screw is used, it will need to be removed before the patient bears weight because of the risk of breaking the screw, although in some centres screw breakage is accepted and the screw left in (this is not our practice). More recently, a suture button technique (Tight-Rope™) has been used and this obviates the need for screw removal.

3 Tri-malleolar fractures. These are always unstable. The posterior malleolar fragment is usually displaced upwards and, if on the lateral X-ray it accounts for one-quarter or more of the articular surface, it needs open reduction and stabilization with a plate or a screw to avoid backward subluxation of the talus. A posterior approach to this fragment and the fibula preserves the more delicate skin laterally. In addition, it is usually

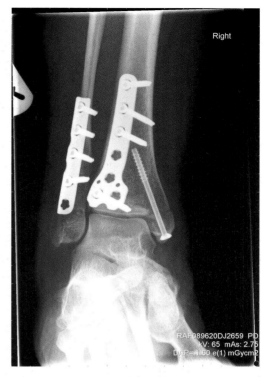

Figure 23.11 Internal fixation of a tri-malleolar fracture. The plate on the tibia is posteriorly applied.

advisable to fix the fibular fracture and the medial malleolus (Fig. 23.11).

Vertical compression fractures

These are most often caused by a fall on the foot from a height. The talus is driven into and shatters the lower end of the tibia; this injury is often known as a Pilon fracture (Fig. 23.12). Management involves stabilizing the bones early with an external fixator which spans the ankle joint to allow the soft tissues to settle. A CT scan is then carried out in order to better define the fracture, and finally a plan is made for definitive management. Thus, the system (which stands for any limb-threatening joint injury) is shown in Box 23.2 below as SPAN, SCAN, PLAN:

This is a severe injury usually leading to stiffness, pain and late arthritic changes.

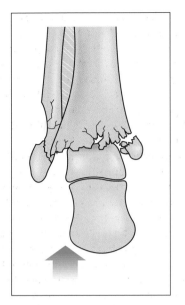

Figure 23.12 Vertical compression fracture—Pilon fracture.

Box 23.2 Limb-threatening joint injury.

SPAN (apply joint spanning external fixator)
SCAN (CT scan to better define the fracture)
PLAN (definitive fixation and rehabilitation)

Rehabilitation

With all these fractures, if the ankle is adequately stabilized by internal fixation, a plaster-cast is not always necessary, but the ideal of early mobilization with non-weight-bearing does require a great deal of patient compliance. Often, therefore, treatment still involves the use of plaster immobilization for protection. Generally, weight-bearing is started at between 2 and 6 weeks, depending on the fracture configuration and casts are usually removed at 6 weeks. Full recovery takes up to a year.

Fractures of the foot

Fractures and dislocations of the talus

Fractures of the body of the talus are rare, but have a poor prognosis for ultimate function because of the associated damage to the ankle articular surface. A CT scan is required to define the fracture and, if there are large displaced fragments, then treatment usually involves ORIF, with great care not to damage the tenuous talar blood supply.

A fracture of the neck of the talus is a serious injury and may occur alone or in combination with a subtalar subluxation (Fig. 23.13). It is

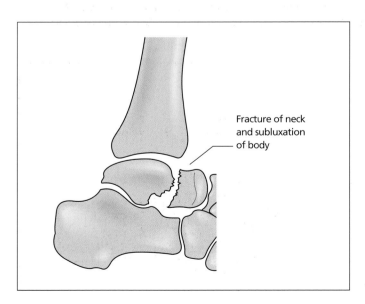

Fracture of neck and subluxation of body

Figure 23.13 Fractured neck of the talus.

usually caused by forced dorsiflexion of the ankle. Accurate reduction by manipulation or open reduction if necessary is essential. Screw or plate fixation aids early motion by stabilizing the fracture. This injury may be complicated by avascular necrosis of the body of the talus due to interruption of the blood supply by the fracture. This is usually evident on X-rays at 8 weeks. Weight-bearing prior to this is therefore not recommended.

Occasionally, the talar neck is fractured and the body completely dislocated from the ankle and subtalar joint. The body is displaced medially and may damage the posterior tibial artery. This injury is frequently open and the risk of avascular necrosis is over 90%. Open reduction is the rule.

Fractures of the calcaneum

These are usually caused by falls from a height onto the heel and are often bilateral. Severity depends on whether the fracture enters the subtalar joint. Because of the way in which the injury occurs, calcaneum fractures are frequently associated with a lumbar spinal burst fracture and all patients must be fully examined with this in mind.

Clinical features
The heel is usually grossly swollen and bruised and the patient is unable to bear weight. Ankle move-ments may be moderately reduced, but subtalar movements are often completely absent.

Fractures of the posterior–superior lip of the calcaneum may still be attached to the Achilles tendon (avulsion fractures) and if lifted up, they need to be reduced and immobilized with the ankle in equinus, or alternatively by internal fixa-tion as a matter of urgency before the skin breaks down ('beak' fracture) (Fig. 23.14).

Fractures involving the subtalar joint usually occur obliquely through the body. The lateral process of the talus acts as a wedge, driving a frag-ment of the posterior articular surface of the sub-talar joint into the body of the calcaneum, causing comminution and 'blowing out' the lateral wall. Lateral X-rays may show flattening of the normal shape of the subtalar joint and diminution of 'Bohler's angle'. An axial projection may be helpful in diagnosing fractures of the sustentaculum and disruption of the subtalar joint (Fig. 23.15). CT scanning is necessary to correctly interpret and treat these injuries.

Treatment
Treatment may be operative or non-operative and to date there is no clear consensus view despite some randomized trials.

Conservative treatment consists of elevation in bed until the swelling subsides, then gradual mobi-lization in a pressure dressing of wool and crêpe

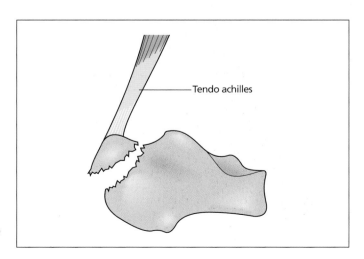

Figure 23.14 Avulsion fracture of the calcaneum.

Tendo achilles

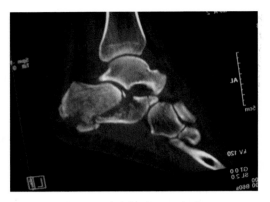

Figure 23.15 CT scan showing fractured calcaneus.

bandage or a light plaster-cast. Weight-bearing is permitted from 6 weeks.

Modern surgical treatment of displaced calcaneal fractures involves a lateral approach, accurate reduction of the large fragments and stabilization with a plate and screws. A cast for 2 weeks precedes non-weight-bearing mobilization and weight-bearing at 6 weeks.

Complications

Occasionally, because of the lateral wall blow out, the peroneal tendons may become trapped between the os calcis and the lateral malleolus and may require surgical release. Damage to the specialized area of fat at the heel pad may give rise to poor coverage and pain. Many patients with sub-talar damage fail to become pain-free and may eventually need a subtalar arthrodesis to restore their ability to walk comfortably.

The proposed advantages of operative reduction (improved heel shape, restoration of articular congruence, reduced likelihood of subtalar and ankle stiffness) may be outweighed by the risks (infection, poor wound healing and sural nerve damage), especially in smokers, non-compliant patients and those with co-morbidities such as diabetes.

Lisfranc injuries

These are rare injuries to the tarsometatarsal joint, usually as a result of rotation of the hindfoot about a fixed forefoot. There may be rupture of the strong plantar ligament which joins the base of the second metatarsal to the medial cuneiform bone (Lisfranc's ligament), or a fracture of one or both of these bones. These fractures are complex and are frequently missed. Early recognition by close inspection of X-rays in a patient with a painful and swollen foot following such a mechanism will result in a more favourable outcome. Recognition is by checking the alignment of the metatarsals to the midfoot bones.

Treatment is by reduction and stabilization (open or closed) with screws or plates.

Fractures of the metatarsals

Basal fractures

Fracture of the base of the fifth metatarsal is common and is caused by an inversion strain of the foot so that the base becomes avulsed by the peroneus brevis tendon.

Treatment

Treatment is with a walking plaster-cast or bandage for 3–6 weeks in the majority of cases. In the special case where the fracture extends into the joint between the fourth and fifth metatarsals (Jones' fractures), treatment is by operative screw stabilization.

Shaft fractures

Metatarsal shaft fractures are common. They are usually caused by crushing and are associated with much soft-tissue damage or swelling.

Treatment

Elevation of the foot, if swollen, is followed by a walking below-knee cast for 6 weeks. If displacement is gross, manipulation and a plaster-cast or open reduction and internal fixation may be necessary, but the soft-tissue insult as a result of the crush may preclude such intervention for weeks or indefinitely.

Stress fractures

These are common fractures, usually of the neck of the second metatarsal, caused by the stress of long periods of walking. They are usually diagnosed when healing, with callus being visible on the X-ray at 3 or 4 weeks.

Treatment

A period of rest from the provocative activity for 6 weeks or so is usually sufficient.

Fractures of the phalanges

These are common injuries and usually of little significance, however, the fracture may interfere with the circulation, necessitating amputation of the toe.

Treatment

They are usually treated by protective dressings, reassurance and allowing the patient to continue walking. Significant displacement on occasions requires reduction and K-wiring to correct deformity.

Infections

Acute infections

Primary infections are uncommon in the ankle and foot except in relation to the toenails which can become in-growing (see below).

Chronic infections

Secondary infections of the joints, especially the MTPJs, from penetrating ulcers of the foot are common in neurological and ischaemic conditions, particularly in diabetes. The forefoot should be X-rayed if a chronic ulcer fails to heal, in order to detect joint destruction or osteomyelitis of the metatarsal heads.

In-growing toenail

The big toe is commonly affected. In cross-section, the edges of the nail curve underneath and the nail 'grows' into the soft tissue. Recurrent infections of the nail fold are common and painful.

Treatment

Antibiotics may cure the severe acute episode, but repeated infections are best treated by removal of either the nail edge or the whole nail. The infection then usually clears, but when the nail re-grows recurrence can occur. The nail may be prevented from re-growing by excision of the germinal matrix (Zadek's procedure). Very careful dissection is necessary to excise the whole of the germinal part of the nail bed. A useful technique consists of resecting the nail and cauterizing the matrix with liquid phenol which denatures the protein of the matrix, thus preventing re-growth.

Tuberculosis

This is uncommon in the ankle or joints of the foot. When it does occur it frequently leads to extensive destruction, necessitating arthrodesis.

Neoplastic conditions

Primary and secondary tumours are uncommon in the ankle and foot. Giant cell tumours are swellings that occur in relation to the tendon sheaths and joints and may resemble ganglia. All swellings which are excised should be sent for histology, irrespective of the macroscopic appearance.

Degenerative conditions

Ankle osteoarthritis

Although taking as much weight as the hip and knee, the ankle is less frequently affected by primary osteoarthritis. Most cases of osteoarthritis are secondary to trauma, injuries of the ankle being very common. Traumatic damage to the articular surface (osteochondral lesions) may predispose to arthritis.

Clinical features

Pain on weight-bearing is the main symptom, and the range of movements gradually diminishes. As the joint space narrows, the talus may tilt within the ankle mortice so that ankle becomes mal-aligned. As in the knee, varus deformity is more common in osteoarthritis (valgus deformity is more often the result of inflammatory joint disease). The characteristic gait pattern is antalgic with the affected limb externally rotated.

Treatment

Disabling pain may require surgery.

1 Arthrodesis is the traditional surgical treatment and gives reasonable function. The ankle is usually fused in about 5 degrees of flexion. Movement is preserved in the subtalar and Chopart's joint which compensate partially for the loss of ankle movement. However, evidence is that these joints may later themselves become arthritic.

2 Arthroplasty. The fact that arthrodesis gives fairly satisfactory results has delayed development of ankle prostheses. Recently though, with new materials and understanding the biomechanics, progress has been made. Several designs are now on the market which are uncemented and have a mobile meniscal bearing to allow for greater freedom of movement. Long-term results are awaited but short-term results are encouraging.

Subtalar osteoarthritis

Osteoarthritis of the subtalar joint may be primary or post-traumatic, usually following os calcis fractures.

Treatment

Activity modification, analgesia and orthoses are the initial management. If this fails to give relief, then surgical treatment is arthrodesis (fusion) of the talus to the os calcis. This gives excellent pain relief but at the cost of permanent stiffness, most notable when walking on uneven terrain. Function overall, however, remains good as the ankle retains all movement.

Talonavicular osteoarthritis

Isolated osteoarthritis of the talonavicular joint is uncommon. In the young it is associated with tarsal coalition. It also occurs in middle age in association with a painful, valgus foot such as occurs with tibialis posterior tendonopathy. Isolated arthrodesis of the talonavicular is the surgical treatment of choice. Triple arthrodesis may be necessary to correct a severe deformity.

Hallux rigidus

Osteoarthritis of the first MTPJ is often called hallux rigidus. This is a common condition, usually occurring in young adults. It is often bilateral and the cause is unknown.

Clinical features

The joint becomes progressively more painful when walking, particularly during the 'push-off' phase. The joint stiffens and, in particular, dorsiflexion is lost, the toe becoming almost rigid. Dorsal osteophytes are often palpable. If there is less stiffness, the term hallux limitus is used. Some compensatory hyper-extension of the interphalangeal joint is usual.

Treatment

Surgery is frequently necessary, and arthrodesis of the joint is the most reliable procedure. In a woman, this limits the height of heel which can be worn, but the procedure gives lasting pain relief. If dorsal osteophytes cause pain due to rubbing on footwear, then these may be removed in a procedure known as a cheilectomy. This, however, does not relieve any deep joint pain which may also be present.

Inflammatory conditions

Rheumatoid arthritis (see Chapter 10)

Clinical features

The ankle and forefoot (MTPJ) are characteristically affected, though any joint may be involved. At the ankle, synovial thickening and gradual destruction of the joint surfaces lead to pain on weight-bearing. The earliest radiological features are a diffuse porosis followed by joint erosions and narrowing. Occasionally, the tarsal joints fuse spontaneously.

The forefoot and toes are often severely deformed, with flexion deformities of the interphalangeal joints leading to clawing. The hindfoot frequently develops a valgus deformity with the posterior tibial tendon becoming defunctional. In the forefoot there is prolapse of the metatarsal heads into the sole as the MTPJs dislocate. This causes metatarsalgia, with the characteristic sensation of walking on pebbles. Hallux valgus is usual and the toes cease to bear weight during walking. These features are sufficiently common in rheumatoid arthritis that patients presenting with severely deformed forefeet should be investigated for the disease.

Treatment

Despite severe deformities, many patients can manage to walk surprisingly well, particularly if the disease is controlled and the shoes are suitably modified.

For the ankle:

1 Synovectomy is less satisfactory than in the knee

2 Fusion may be necessary, particularly in the young, but in a generalized joint condition, any procedure which increases stiffness leads to poor function

3 Ankle joint replacement maintains some motion and helps with pain.

For the hindfoot, fusion of isolated joints for pain and deformity often help. In a severe case with deformity, triple arthrodesis may be helpful.

Forefoot surgery aims to reduce pain and prevent ulcers forming over areas of pressure. Clawing of the toes, with pressure from the shoes on the flexed interphalangeal joint, may require either excision of the proximal phalanges or interphalangeal fusions. Symptoms caused by overload under the metatarsal heads may be treated by shortening, angled osteotomies (Weil osteotomies) or more traditionally by excision of the metatarsal heads,

together with an ellipse of skin from the ball of the foot. When this excised wound is closed, the toes are drawn down. The first metatarsal may be fused at the MTPJ or the head may be excised (Kates–Kessel–Kay operation).

Gout

This condition characteristically affects the first MTPJ (95% of cases are men). Acute attacks of severe pain with swelling and erythema are usual. The joint is gradually destroyed and develops secondary osteoarthritis.

Treatment

This is by drug therapy (see Chapter 10).

Ischaemia

Arterial disease is common in the ageing population. Lower limb ischaemia may manifest itself as intermittent claudication or by the development of gangrene of the toes, or both. Microvascular disease is common in diabetics who may present with ulceration.

Diabetic neuropathy may also be associated with disintegration of the joints of the foot, with collapse and increasing deformity (Charcot's neuroarthropathy). Secondary ulceration may then occur. This is a difficult condition to manage, but short periods of cast immobilization may delay progression. Purpose-designed footwear may help to prevent many of these complications.

Neurological conditions

Examples of such neurological conditions which affect the foot and ankle are:

1 Hereditary motor sensory neuropathies, e.g. Charcot–Marie–Tooth disease

2 Friedreich's ataxia

3 Spina bifida

4 Poliomyelitis.

Chapter 24

Orthopaedic techniques

Operative procedures

Joint aspiration

Aspiration of a joint is usually carried out for diagnostic purposes. It will distinguish between synovial fluid (effusion), pus (pyarthrosis) or blood (haemarthrosis). An infected joint may contain fluid which is somewhat turbid due to the presence of white cells, or frank pus which is thick and creamy and composed largely of white cells and debris, usually with many organisms. Blood in a joint does not normally clot and may still be aspirated several days after bleeding. In appropriate cases, the synovial fluid may be examined for urate or pyrophosphate crystals.

Technique

The risk of introducing organisms is considerable, so any procedure which involves introducing a needle into a joint should be carried out with full sterile precautions, with the limb draped and the operator gowned and masked.

General anaesthesia may be used, or local infiltration anaesthesia may be preferred. Lidocaine is a suitable local anaesthetic and after infiltration of

Lecture Notes: Orthopaedics and Fractures, 4e.
By T Duckworth and CM Blundell. Published 2010 by Blackwell Publishing.

the skin, the deep tissues and particularly the synovium should be well infiltrated. Inflamed synovium is very sensitive and difficult to anaesthetize adequately.

For the aspiration, a wide-bore needle is usually used, attached to a 20–50-ml syringe.

The knee and hip joint require aspiration most frequently.

The knee

This joint will usually be distended and easy to enter. The needle is most easily introduced close to the medial border of the patella near the upper margin. The point should be directed downwards and towards the centre of the joint, with care to avoid the articular cartilage. A definite resistance will be felt as the synovium is entered. After complete aspiration, the joint is wrapped in a Robert Jones pressure bandage of alternate layers of crêpe bandage and wool.

The hip

Passing a needle into the hip is more difficult because of the depth of the joint. Two techniques are possible. The centre of the head of the femur lies directly under the 'mid-inguinal point' and behind the femoral artery. The needle is inserted 2 cm lateral to the pulsation of the artery and directed backwards and medially.

Alternatively, a long needle may be introduced laterally at the tip of the greater trochanter and passed along the upper surface of the neck into the joint. If the joint is not distended, only 2 or 3 ml of fluid may be aspirated. Frequently hip aspiration is carried out under ultrasound guidance by a musculoskeletal radiologist.

Biopsy

Biopsy is used to obtain specimens of tissues for histological examination or culture.

Needle biopsy

This is occasionally useful for small specimens of tissue, e.g. from the spine or bone marrow. The specimen may, however, be inadequate or unrepresentative of the whole lesion.

Punch biopsy

This more sophisticated technique uses a punch introduced through a cannula. Its main use in orthopaedic work is to take samples of iliac crest bone, usually for the diagnosis of metabolic bone disease. It can give an adequate core of bone with little trauma and without the need for a full exposure. A similar technique is used for bone marrow aspiration, usually from the sternum. With radiological control, specimens can be taken from the spine and paraspinal tissues.

Surgical biopsy

This is the preferred technique for tumours of soft tissue and bone. With small lesions, excision biopsy may be possible, including an adequate margin of normal tissue.

The piece of tissue should be large enough to be representative, should avoid necrotic tissue and should, if possible, contain some normal tissue. This is particularly important with pleomorphic tumours such as osteosarcomata. Biopsy of suspected malignant neoplasms should always be carried out after discussion with the definitive centre treating the tumour, such as a regional sarcoma unit (see Chapter 12, p. 93).

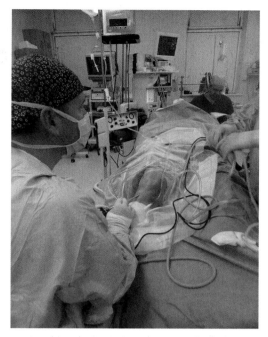

Figure 24.1 Knee arthroscopy.

Arthroscopy

This procedure has steadily developed over the last 15–20 years with improved optical techniques. The modern instrument is similar in principle to the cystoscope and uses fibre-optic illumination (Fig. 24.1). The instrument is passed into the joint through a small skin incision under local or general anaesthesia. The telescope fits inside a cannula introduced through the capsule and synovium with a sharp trocar.

The knee has received most attention, but techniques have been developed for examination and surgery of many joints, notably the shoulder, ankle, wrist, hip and small joints of the fingers. There is also increasing interest in performing spinal surgery with similar minimally invasive techniques.

In the knee, it is possible to see all the important structures, including almost the whole of both menisci, the cruciates and the articular cartilage. Biopsy of the synovial membrane is possible, using special forceps introduced through the trocar, and minor operative procedures may be carried out in this way. Techniques have been developed to enable

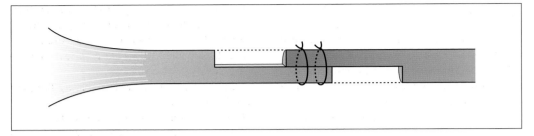

Figure 24.2 Tendon lengthening by Z plasty.

elaborate operations to be carried out. It is possible to excise fragments of damaged tissue, e.g. from the articular surfaces or menisci, to repair menisci and ligaments, to remove loose bodies and to pin osteocartilaginous fragments into position. Extensive synovectomy is possible, as is ligament repair and replacement. The operating instruments are introduced through small stab incisions or 'portals' and the procedure is viewed through the arthroscope. The use of a small television camera attached to the arthroscope is standard practice and is a valuable teaching aid. The technique requires considerable skill and experience, but results, particularly in terms of rapid rehabilitation, can be very good.

Soft-tissue release

This is an operative technique designed to correct deformity caused by soft-tissue contracture. It is used for the correction of such conditions as club foot and the deformities associated with paralytic conditions.

The skin may be involved in the contracture and the incision may have to be planned to allow skin elongation.

Tight soft tissues are then released systematically, including fascia, tendons, capsule, etc. Frequently, tendon lengthening alone is sufficient, e.g. the tendo achilles for an equinus deformity of the ankle. Nerves and vessels may be the ultimate limiting factor. A period in a plaster-cast is usually necessary to maintain correction.

Tenotomy

This means dividing a tendon, usually to correct a soft-tissue contracture. The procedure may be

carried out 'closed', by using a fine knife introduced through the skin. This procedure is dangerous for deeply placed or inaccessible tendons and in these cases the tendon is lengthened by an 'open' operation. If the tendon is to be lengthened and resutured, this is usually done by a 'Z' technique (Fig. 24.2).

Tendon transfer

Paralytic muscular imbalance may lead to joint contractures in the growing child. Tendon transfer may be used to restore the balance or occasionally to restore a specific function, e.g. in the hand.

The best results are obtained when:

1 The muscle whose tendon is to be transferred has full power and is under voluntary control
2 The tendon is only transferred a short distance, e.g. a lateral transfer of the tibialis anterior to correct a varus deformity of the foot (transfers through the interosseous membranes are usually less successful)
3 The muscle works in the same phase as the group it is meant to reinforce, e.g. a flexor tendon to replace a flexor
4 The tendon can be implanted firmly into bone under tension.

The wrist flexors can often be spared to replace non-functioning finger or thumb tendons, e.g. flexor carpi ulnaris to replace the long finger flexors. Re-education is quickly achieved.

The tibialis anterior or posterior and the peronei are frequently used to correct inversion or eversion imbalance in the foot.

Osteotomy

This means dividing a bone, usually by open operation (osteoclasis means fracturing a bone).

It is used to correct bone deformity and occasionally persistent joint contracture. In the latter case, it should be done as near to the joint as possible. All types of deformity can be corrected, including rotation.

The osteotomy is allowed to unite either with external plaster fixation or by internal fixation. There are many osteotomies for specific purposes, e.g. through the innominate bone to restore acetabular alignment (Salter operation) or through the os calcis to correct inversion of the heel in a club foot (Dwyer operation).

Osteotomy has also been used to relieve pain in osteoarthritis of the hip and knee. At the hip the bone is divided just above the lesser trochanter (McMurray technique), and at the knee through the upper tibia. The osteotomies are allowed to unite in the usual way. Pain relief is usually immediate if the procedure has been successful. The mechanism of action is unknown though mechanical realignment is the probable mechanism.

Arthrotomy

This term simply means opening a joint surgically to secure drainage or to carry out an exploration or surgical procedure.

Arthrodesis

Surgical fusion of a joint is known as arthrodesis. (Ankylosis means spontaneous fusion, e.g. following a joint infection.) Arthrodesis is usually performed for one of two reasons:

1 For pain relief in a joint which has been severely damaged by disease

2 To stabilize a joint which has lost its stability because of ligamentous damage or paralysis. The joint may be fused either by:

- Clearing the articular surfaces of cartilage, bringing the raw surfaces together, and holding the position until bony union occurs, or
- An extra-articular technique where the fusion by-passes the joint, e.g. the Britten technique for

hip fusion (now rarely used). Extra-articular fusion used to be popular for fusing tuberculous joints. In many cases, when the disease was cured, the joint itself would then fuse by bony ankylosis.

Many techniques are used for fixing the joint until fusion occurs:

1 External splintage, usually plaster of Paris

2 A combination of external fixation with compression, e.g. the Charnley fusion of the knee, where the condyles are cut off squarely and the cancellous ends held firmly together by an external compression clamp

3 Internal fixation by screws, plates or rods, etc, e.g. plate fixation of the metatarsophalangeal joint (Fig. 24.3) or rod fixation of a scoliosis.

4 Fusion may be assisted by bone grafting, e.g. fusion of the spine may be performed anteriorly by excising the intervertebral disc and putting a graft across the gap, or posteriorly by rawing the posterior bony elements and packing with iliac bone

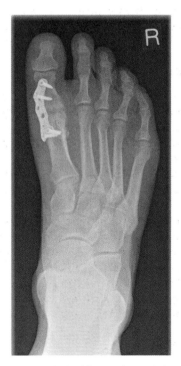

Figure 24.3 Arthrodesis of first metatarsophalangeal joint with plate fixation.

chips or a large cortico-cancellous bone graft cut to fit around the spinous processes.

Whatever technique is used, protection is necessary for a long period; usually at least 3 months, and success is more likely if the joint is already stiff before starting.

Arthroplasty

Artificial joint replacement has received much attention over the last two decades, and solutions have been found for many of the engineering and biological problems, only for these to be replaced by other and more subtle problems as experience of the technique grows.

The hip and knee have received most attention and very satisfactory function can be attained with modern techniques.

There are basically three types of arthroplasty.

Excision arthroplasty

The joint surfaces are excised completely or partially. Fibrous tissue forms across the gap, giving some stability. Many materials have been interfaced between the joint surfaces to allow better movement, e.g. deep fascia, silastic sheets or flexible connectors, plastic laminae, etc. This type of arthroplasty usually has the disadvantage of incomplete pain relief coupled with instability and is now usually regarded as a 'rescue' procedure following failure of a joint replacement.

Hemi-arthroplasty

Only one of the joint surfaces is replaced, e.g. hemi-arthroplasty of the hip for intracapsular fractures (see Fig. 21.14). This is satisfactory if one joint surface is in good condition, e.g. following a fracture, but rarely in osteoarthritis.

Total arthroplasty

Both joint surfaces are replaced, either with metal entirely or metal or ceramic bearing against plastic, usually high-density polyethylene. These have the advantage of giving good function, but are vulnerable to sepsis or mechanical failure, which may loosen or otherwise destroy them.

Principles

Current ideas on replacement arthroplasty suggest certain principles.

1 The combination of stainless steel, titanium or cobalt-chrome for one component and high-density polyethylene for the other appears to give the best combination of low friction and good wear properties. Ceramic prostheses are gaining popularity for use in the young due to their excellent wear characteristics.

2 The articular surface should allow for adequate movement in the required directions whilst restraining movement in unwanted directions, to the extent that this is not prevented by ligaments damaged by disease.

3 The prosthesis should be bonded to bone either by using acrylic cement or it may be coated (with a substance such as hydroxyapatite) or covered in a 'sintered' material into which bone can grow.

4 The operative procedure should be designed to reduce the risk of infection to a minimum.

5 If failure occurs, it should be possible to remove the prosthesis, and, if necessary, perform an arthrodesis or a further joint replacement, which might be possible if enough bone stock is maintained. Specific implants have been designed for revision joint replacement.

Replacement of individual joints is considered in the appropriate chapters.

Laminectomy

The term strictly means an approach to the spinal canal by removing the laminae of one or more vertebrae with the intervening ligaments. The procedure may be carried out on one side only, or bilaterally, in which case the spinous processes and ligaments are removed. It is often possible to remove a prolapsed intervertebral disc by making an opening through the ligamentum flavum and nibbling away a little of the laminae above and below. This is often called a laminectomy, but should strictly be called a 'laminotomy' or 'fenestration'.

Amputation

It may be necessary to amputate part of a limb for one of the following reasons:

1 Its retention may threaten life, e.g. neoplasia, 'crush' syndrome, severe infection, etc.

2 It is non-viable, e.g. following trauma, vascular insufficiency, etc.

3 Function or appearance could be improved by replacement of the part with a suitable prosthesis, e.g. congenital or paralytic deformities

4 Pain which is resistant to other forms of therapy. This is an unusual reason for amputation and if the pain is severe and well-established, amputation may fail to relieve the symptoms, with persistence of phantom pain.

The commonest reason for amputation in Western society is ischaemia due to vascular disease. Reasons for amputation are summarized in Box 24.1.

Whenever amputation is considered, the fullest cooperation with an experienced prosthetist is required, both before and after surgery.

Having decided that amputation is the procedure of choice, the level should be decided to give the best possible function and appearance consistent with removing the pathology. If the amputation is required to eliminate a neoplasm, there will usually be little choice of level, this depending on the need to remove the tumour completely. It is usually necessary to amputate through the joint above the pathology or even higher, and this may result in a stump which gives less than optimum function.

Where such considerations do not apply, the level can often be decided on functional grounds, the 'sites of election' for various levels having been worked out from long experience. The normal considerations, in general terms, are:

1 The more peripheral the amputation, the better, except that for any given level, a stump which is too long may make the fitting of an adequate prosthesis just below it very difficult or impossible

2 If the elbow or knee joints can be retained, function is very much improved

3 For most lower-limb amputations, very adequate functional prostheses can be provided, but the higher the amputation, the more difficult this becomes

4 Prosthetic function for upper limb amputations is relatively poor because of the complicated demands of hand function and the difficulty of replacing sensibility

5 The psychological preparation for amputation is very important and, indeed, amputation should usually be regarded as only a stage in a long-term programme of rehabilitation.

Lower-limb amputation

Amputation of toes

This is frequently necessary for trauma and deformity. It is rarely followed by significant functional loss, although the big toe plays a significant part in normal walking.

Occasionally, with penetrating ulcers, particularly in diabetes, it may be necessary to amputate a toe with its associated metatarsal ray. The gap closes and can give a good functional foot.

Amputation through the forefoot

This is also usually performed for trauma or occasionally in diabetic ischaemia. It is not suitable for ischaemia due to large vessel disease. It can give good function, the shoe having to be padded.

Amputation through the mid-tarsal region

This is usually best avoided as, depending on the level, the stump may become deformed by the unopposed action of the tibialis muscles, the peronei having been sectioned.

Amputation through the ankle

This is known as a Symes amputation. In this procedure, the os calcis and talus are shelled out of the heel, the skin of which is then used as a flap to

---

Box 24.1 Reasons for amputation.

- Life-threatening   DEADLY
- Non-viable limb   DEAD
- Poor function   DEBILITATING

---

cover the tibia and fibula, with the malleoli removed at the same level. This gives a satisfactory end-bearing stump. It is usually carried out for deformity or trauma. The prosthesis consists of a hinged foot on a shell which is designed to fit around the prominence of the ankle. It has the advantage of being capable of load-bearing without a prosthesis.

Trans-tibial amputation

This is one of the commonest amputations and the indications are many. There has been a definite trend in vascular surgery to attempt a below-knee (trans-tibial) rather than the traditional above-knee (trans-femoral) amputation because of the much better function which can be obtained if the knee is preserved, particularly in the elderly. The optimal site for tibial section is usually considered to be 17 cm below the knee, but a stump as short as 7 cm can be fitted, albeit with a less satisfactory prosthesis. Traditionally, the fibula is divided 2 cm higher, but the technique of osteomyoplastic amputation divides the fibula at the same level as the tibia, and a periosteal tube is used to form a firm bridge between the two ends.

Equal anterior and posterior flaps are usually used, but in vascular disease a longer posterior flap of skin and muscle is recommended.

The most satisfactory prosthesis is the patellar-tendon-bearing limb, which fits closely around the upper tibia and takes most weight on the patellar tendon. The end of the stump does not normally bear weight. With this type of prosthesis, if fitted correctly, an above-knee harness is not required. The overall cosmesis can be very satisfactory.

Mid-thigh amputation

This level of amputation is frequently needed for ischaemia and trauma. Function is less satisfactory than with trans-tibial amputations. The stump should be as long as possible, but allowing 12 cm between the end and the position of the knee hinge of a prosthesis. This has a bucket top which fits the stump closely, much of the weight-bearing being taken through the ischial tuberosity. A well-fitted prosthesis can give a very satisfactory gait.

Through-the-hip and hindquarter amputations

These amputations are usually performed for neoplasia. They are mutilating and difficult to fit with a functional prosthesis.

Upper-limb amputation

Amputations of the finger and thumb

These amputations are almost always performed for trauma. Fingers are usually most effectively amputated through the joints. As much length as possible should be preserved, provided that the joints are not stiff. If the whole index is lost, it is best to amputate through the second metacarpal to avoid an ugly metacarpal stump. The function of the index is readily taken over by the middle finger. The little finger contributes considerably to the normal power grip. If it is amputated, it may be useful to preserve the head of the metacarpal as this widens the hand.

The thumb is the most important digit and as much length as possible should be preserved, even if it is stiff. The metacarpal alone can give reasonable function. If the whole thumb is lost, it is possible to reconstruct it, either by rotating the second metacarpal to 'pollicize' the index, or by replacing the thumb with a bone graft and tube pedicle graft. In this case it is necessary to provide an island of sensation, by using an innervated pedicle from another digit. Without sensibility, function of the thumb is greatly reduced.

Amputations through the forearm and upper arm

The elbow should be preserved if possible as its movements may be useful in powering a hand prosthesis, usually a double hook or specialized prosthesis. If the elbow is amputated, the prosthesis is powered by shoulder movements acting through a series of straps and functional capacity is very limited. A cosmetic hand is provided when function is not needed. If the other arm and hand are normal, many patients prefer not to bother with a powered prosthesis.

Attempts are now being made to provide external power and some form of sensibility to improve upper limb prostheses.

Amputation through the shoulder and forequarter

As in the lower limb, these are usually needed for neoplasia. If the upper end of the humerus can be preserved, this gives a better cosmetic appearance to the shoulder. Even preservation of the scapula alone gives a tolerable appearance, but the forequarter amputation is extremely unsightly and very difficult to fit with an adequate prosthesis, which is usually only for cosmesis.

Amputations in children

These present special problems in that the bones continue to grow if the amputation is through the shafts and the ends may ulcerate through the skin, necessitating re-amputation.

Amputations through the joints avoid this problem and are to be preferred. Children adapt very rapidly to below-knee amputation.

Amputation of the upper limbs for congenital malformation should usually be deferred until the child's function is assessed, as even the most severe deformities can be compatible with good function. If the child has one normal arm, a functional prosthesis on the other side is usually completely ignored.

Non-operative techniques and appliances

Manipulation of fractures and dislocations

Muscular relaxation is usually necessary for a successful manipulation. This can be achieved by one of the following techniques.

1 Carrying out the manipulation quickly and unexpectedly. This technique is useful for the reduction of finger joints and elbow dislocations. It obviously requires confidence and skill and only one attempt is usually possible.

2 Heavy sedation, e.g. with a short-acting benzodiazepine. This has the advantage of avoiding possible complications of a general or local anaesthetic, but rarely allows sufficient relaxation for a difficult manipulation.

3 Local anaesthesia. This may be obtained either by direct infiltration of the site, e.g. the fracture haematoma block, or by regional nerve or venous block. The former carries the small theoretical risk of infecting the fracture site, but both techniques usually relieve muscle spasm as well as pain. These techniques are particularly useful in the emergency department setting or where the patient is unfit.

4 General anaesthesia.

The manipulative technique usually consists of working out the mechanism by which the displacement has occurred and reversing this mechanism. It is often necessary to disimpact the fragments by traction and over-riding may need to be corrected by increasing the angulation at the fracture site, then 'hitching' the ends. Difficulties may arise when soft tissues, such as muscle or fascia, are interposed between the fragments. In these cases, there is usually an obvious block to reduction and the skin and soft tissues may be dimpled inwards by the attempt. When this happens, open reduction is usually necessary to extract the soft tissues. Forcible manipulation is rarely necessary and may cause serious injury to important soft tissues.

Splintage

In an emergency, e.g. at the roadside, splints can be improvised from anything available, such as rolled-up newspapers, an umbrella, etc. The upper limb is easily splinted by making up a simple sling. The lower limb can be splinted by tying the legs together. It is usually best to put the limb gently into a neutral position if it is severely angulated following a fracture.

Types of splint

Splints made from polythene, wire mesh, padded wood and plaster of Paris are in widespread use. They are usually bandaged in position, care being taken not to apply them too tightly and to avoid

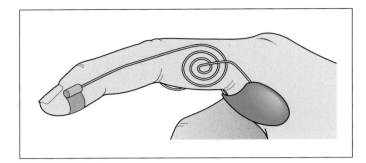

Figure 24.4 Lively finger splint.

pressure on prominences and superficial nerves. The lateral popliteal nerve at the knee is particularly vulnerable.

Functional splints

These splints may be prescribed to control certain movements, whilst still allowing or encouraging function, e.g. various types of spring-loaded or 'lively' splints are available for the hand, usually to encourage finger movements and to avoid contractures (Fig. 24.4).

Slings

Two types of sling are in regular use.

1 Broad sling, made from a triangular bandage. This is used when the weight of the whole limb requires support, e.g. a fracture of the clavicle or a dislocation of the shoulder.

2 Collar and cuff, designed to support the elbow in flexion whilst allowing the weight of the arm to exert traction, e.g. on a fracture of the humeral shaft. It is usually the most comfortable sling for a severely swollen elbow.

Plaster of Paris technique

Plaster of Paris made from gypsum is the most widely used material for fashioning external splints. It can be used in several ways.

1 Simple splint. The limbs or joints are placed in the desired position and the splint is fashioned by laying wet plaster in strips to form a half-plaster or 'gutter' splint. A better fit can be obtained by making a complete circumferential plaster and cutting this into two halves longitudinally (bi-

valved). Both halves can then be used individually or together.

2 Complete plaster-cast. The type and extent of the cast will depend on the immobilization required, e.g. half-leg, full-leg, etc. Plaster-casts which immobilize the hip or shoulder are usually known as 'spicas' and their application requires considerable experience if they are to be comfortable (Fig. 24.5).

As a general rule, to immobilize a fracture adequately, the joints above and below need to be incorporated in the plaster. This rule may be broken if the fracture is very close to the end of a long bone, e.g. a Colles' fracture.

3 Functional cast, e.g. by the incorporation of hinges or springs. This technique allows greater function in the joints with less stiffness.

4 Plaster bed. In this the patient can lie for long periods without developing pressure sores, the plaster being made to conform to his/her contours. These are now rarely used.

Application of plaster of Paris

The routine use of plaster of Paris requires considerable skill and attention to detail, but every doctor should be capable of applying a simple cast to immobilize a fracture.

It is usual nowadays to use ready-prepared plaster bandages which are reliable and predictable in their setting. Everything should be assembled before starting to apply the plaster, as the setting time is short.

1 The amount of protection for the limb depends on the circumstances. If swelling is present or

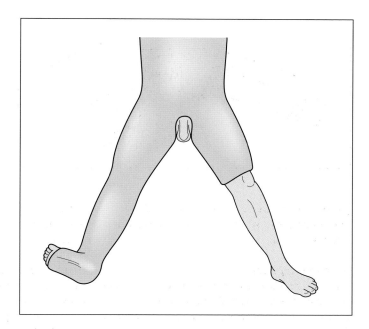

Figure 24.5 Hip spica.

expected, some padding is necessary, usually a single layer of plaster wool wrapped evenly round the limb, paying particular attention to pressure points and prominences. If swelling is unlikely to be a problem, the plaster may be applied unpadded and skin-tight. This gives good immobilization, but is dangerous if applied incorrectly and is difficult to remove. This problem may be partly overcome by applying a stretch stockinette sleeve to the limb before applying the plaster.

2 The roll of plaster is soaked in lukewarm water in a bucket until bubbles begin to emerge from the ends of the roll. Surplus water is then gently squeezed out and the bandage rolled onto the limb, without applying any tension and carefully avoiding folds and wrinkles. The plaster is rubbed to distribute the material evenly between layers and finally smoothed off. An assistant may be needed to hold the limb in the correct position, but he/she should be careful to avoid pressure with his/her fingers on the cast until it is set. The plaster wool or stockinette may be folded over the ends of the cast to give a neat comfortable finish.

3 The cast dries within 5–10 minutes, but is not fully hard until 24 hours later during which time weight bearing should be avoided.

> **Box 24.2** Complications of cast usage.
>
> - Occlusion of the circulation. If the limb is likely to swell considerably, especially acute limb trauma such as a tibial fracture, the patient is best kept under observation
> - Nerve palsies due to pressure
> - Pressure sores—often signalled by staining of the cast or by smell
> - Occasionally, patients in a hip spica develop paralytic ileus, with vomiting and collapse. This can usually be cured by splitting or removing the plaster

4 The patient should be given printed instructions to watch for changes in the circulation and sensation in the limb, and to return if the cast is uncomfortable, tight or rubbing the skin.

Complications of case usage are listed in Box 24.2.

If there is any suggestion that a plaster is too tight, it should be split with a plaster saw and the opening spread. If this is done, the split should be made down to the skin throughout the whole length of the plaster.

A fracture which is not in correct alignment may be improved by wedging the plaster. This involves

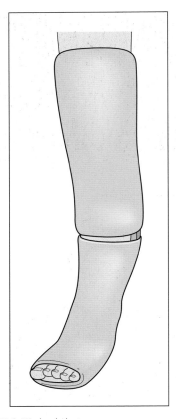

Figure 24.6 Wedged plaster.

making a cut around half the circumference and wedging the opening with a wooden block. If the X-ray is then satisfactory, the plaster may be completed again (Fig. 24.6).

Synthetic casting materials

See Chapter 5.

Traction

See Chapter 5.

Braces and supports

The design of splints, braces and other externally applied appliances is known as orthotics and the appliances themselves as orthoses.

An orthopaedic appliance is usually used to hold a joint or a limb to:

1 Relieve pain

2 Allow a fracture to unite by relieving stresses

3 Compensate for weakness of muscles, ligaments or bones during weight-bearing or other functions.

Common types of appliance in the management of fractures and dislocations

Thomas splint

This is discussed in Chapter 5 (Fig. 5.3, p. 36). It was devised by Hugh Owen Thomas as a knee splint. It is now mainly used for femoral shaft fractures and has the advantage that the patient can be moved with the splint in position. Its application is straightforward, but attention to detail is necessary if complications are to be avoided.

1 The splint is selected by measuring the circumference of the upper thigh at groin level to give the ring size. The length should be that of the good leg from crotch to sole of foot, plus 15–23 cm.

2 The splint is prepared by covering it with three slings made from non-stretch bandage or commercially available Velcro slings, one under the thigh, one under the knee and one just above the Achilles tendon.

3 The limb is shaved, the fracture manipulated, and the skin traction applied on each side, with felt pads over the malleoli to prevent pressure. A crêpe bandage then holds the extensions in place.

4 The tapes are tied over the end of the splint, the outer one going over the lateral bar and the inner one under it to counteract the tendency of the limb to rotate externally. Pads and small aluminium 'gutter' splints may be used under the thigh to secure the correct position of the fracture.

5 If the splint is to be on for a long period, it may be suspended by overhead slings and a weight may be attached to the end to relieve the groin pressure.

6 The splint may be used with skeletal traction through the tibia, but a knee flexion piece is then needed and the principle of fixed traction no longer applies.

This device is used for supporting the leg in the elevated position. Its use is self-explanatory. The leg is usually on traction (see Fig. 5.8).

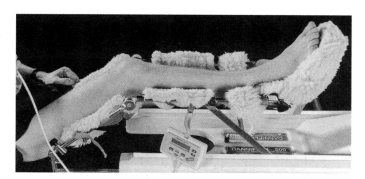

Figure **24.7** Continuous passive motion machine.

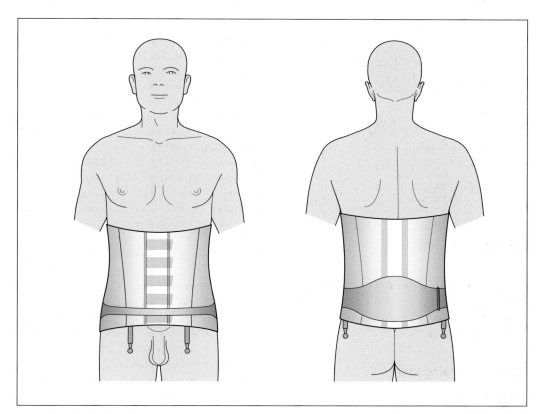

Figure 24.8 Lumbosacral support.

Continuous passive motion frame

This device incorporates an electric motor to flex and extend the joint to be moved. Movement is achieved passively with a slow and controlled rhythm and the range can be adjusted as the movement improves. It is particularly useful following knee arthroplasty (Fig. 24.7).

Lumbosacral support or corset

Many types are available. They are usually made of canvas with steel inserts or of block leather and aluminium, or more recently of polythene and plastazote. They are made either by moulding directly on to the patient (Fig. 24.8) or on to a plaster-cast.

Cervical collar

This is useful for the relief of pain in acute conditions or spondylosis, or for immobilization of injuries. Many types are available.

1 Polystyrene type, which can be cut to size and held with Velcro. It is valuable and reliable for short-term use.

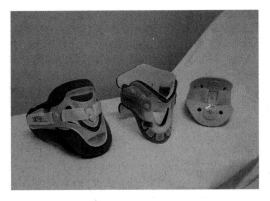

Figure 24.9 Types of cervical collar.

2 Fully-shaped collar, made from polythene and foam-lined. This may be made adjustable (Fig. 24.9).

Splints can be used to control joints in paralytic conditions or following ligamentous or bony damage.

1 Full leg caliper to control knee, ankle and foot, with stops entering the heel of the shoe. This may be supplied with a lockable knee hinge to allow sitting.

2 Below-knee calipers to control ankle or foot movements. These may have a single iron on one side or a double iron. A widely used example is the inside iron with a T-strap around the ankle, usually to control varus or valgus instability (Fig. 24.10). The trend is towards calipers which are lighter and more cosmetically acceptable, and fibre-glass and moulded polythene splints can be used for many conditions. A polythene foot drop splint is one example of an ankle–foot orthoses (Fig. 24.11).

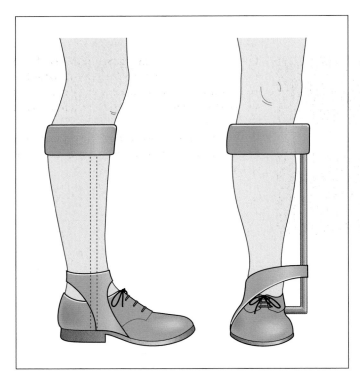

Figure 24.10 T-strap and inside iron.

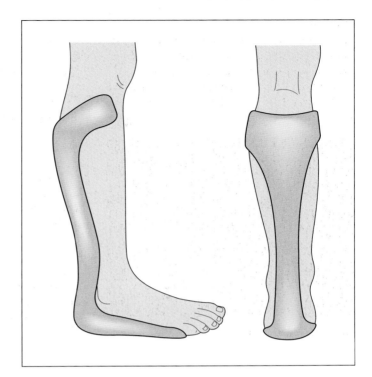

Figure 24.11 Foot drop splint.

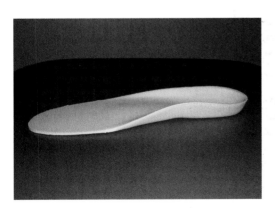

Figure 24.12 An in-shoe orthosis.

3 Arch supports and metatarsal supports. These in-shoe orthoses are moulded to suit the condition to be treated, e.g. a metatarsal support provides for weight-bearing behind the metatarsal heads (Fig. 24.12).

4 Walking appliances. Many types are in use: axillary and elbow crutches, walking frames, rollators, etc (Fig. 24.13).

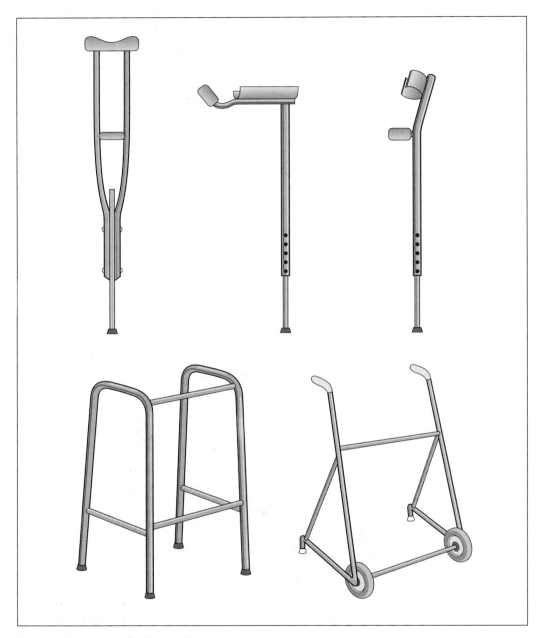

Figure 24.13 A range of walking appliances.

Appendix

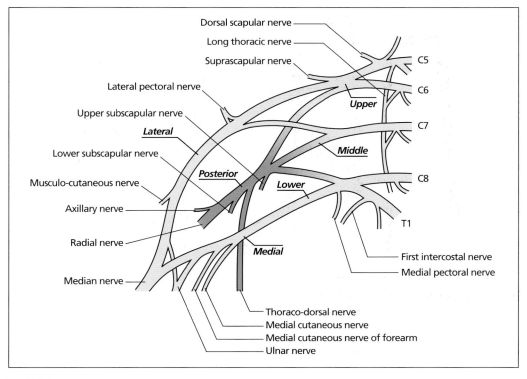

Brachial plexus

Appendix

Muscles of principal importance supplied by the major nerves

Accessory nerve	C3, 4	Trapezius
Thoraco-dorsal nerve	C5, 7, 8	Latissimus dorsi
Dorsal scapular nerve	C4, 5	Rhomboids
Lateral pectoral nerve	C5, 6, 7	Pectoralis major
Medial pectoral nerve	C8, T1	Pectoralis minor
Long thoracic nerve	C5, 6, 7	Serratus anterior
Axillary nerve	C5, 6	Deltoid, teres minor
Sub-scapular nerves	C5, 6, 7	Subscapularis, teres major
Supra-scapular nerve	C4, 5, 6	Supra-spinatus, infra-spinatus
Musculo-cutaneous nerve	C5, 6, 7	Coraco-brachialis, biceps, brachialis (C6, 7)
Median nerve	C5, 6, 7, 8, T1	Pronator teres (C6)
		Flexor carpi radialis (C6, 7)
		Palmaris longus (C7, 8)
		Flexor carpi ulnaris (C7, 8)
		Flexor digitorum superficialis (C7, 8, T1)
		Flexor pollicis longus (C8, T1)
		Flexor digitorum profundus (C8, T1)
		Pronator quadratus (C8, T1)
		Abd. pollicis brevis
		Opponens pollicis
		Flexor pollicis brevis
		Lateral 2 lumbricals (C8, T1)
Ulnar nerve		Flexor carpi ulnaris (C7, 8)
		Flexor digitorum profundus (C8, T1)
	C7, 8, T1	Flexor pollicis brevis
		Adductor pollicis (C8, T1)
		Palmaris brevis
		Hypothenar muscles, interossei, medial two lumbricals (C8, T1)
Radial nerve	C5, 6, 7, 8, T1	Triceps (C6, 7, 8)
		Brachio-radialis (C5, 6)
		Extensor carpi radialis longus and brevis (C6, 7)
		Extensor digitorum (C7, 8)
		Ext. dig. minimi (C7)
		Extensor carpi ulnaris (C7, 8)
		Supinator (C5, 6)
		Abd. pollicis longus (C7, 8)
		Ext. pollicis brevis (C7, 8)
		Ext. pollicis longus (C7, 8)
		Ext. pollicis indicis (C7, 8)
First lumbar nerve	L1	Psoas minor
Second and third lumbar nerves	L1, 2 (3)	Psoas, major, iliacus
Obturator nerve	L2, 3, 4	Gracilis (L2, 3)
		Adductor longus (L2, 3, 4)
		Adductor brevis (L2, 3, 4)
		Adductor magnus (L3, 4 + sciatic)
		Obturator externus (L2, 3, 4)
Femoral nerve	L2, 3, 4	Sartorius (L2, 3)
		Quadriceps (L2, 3, 4)
		Pectineus (L2, 3)
Superior gluteal nerve	L4, 5, S1	Gluteus medius, gluteus minimus, tensor, fasciae latae

Inferior gluteal nerve	L5, S1, 2	Gluteus maximus
Sciatic nerve	L4, 5, S1, 2, 3	Add. magnus (L4, 5 + obturator)
		Biceps femoris (L5, S1, 2, 3)
Sciatic tibial division		Semitendinosus (L5, S1, 2)
		Semi-membranosus (L5, S1, 2)
		Biceps (S1, 2, 3)
		Gastrocnemius (S1, 2)
		Soleus (S1, 2)
		Plantaris (S1, 2)
		Popliteus (L4, 5, S1)
		Flexor hallucis longus (S2, 3)
		Flexor digitorum longus (S2, 3)
		Tibialis posterior (L4, 5)
		Plantar muscles (S2, 3)
Sciatic, common peroneal		Biceps (L5, S1)
		Tibialis anterior (L4, 5)
		Extensor hallucis longus (L5, S1)
		Extensor digitorum longus, peroneus tertius (L5, S1)
		Peroneus longus, peroneus brevis (L5, S1)
		Extensor digitorum brevis (S1, 2)

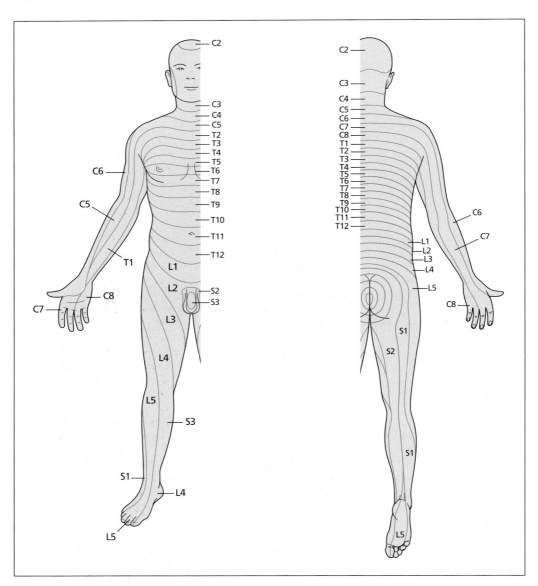

Sensory dermatomes

Index

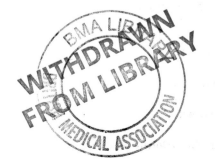